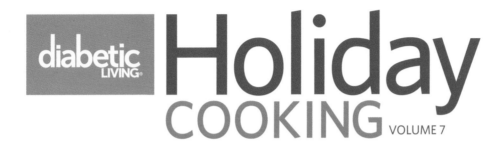

diabetic LIVING Holiday COOKING VOLUME 7

DIABETIC LIVING® HOLIDAY COOKING IS PART
OF A BOOK SERIES PUBLISHED BY BETTER
HOMES AND GARDENS SPECIAL
INTEREST MEDIA, DES MOINES, IOWA

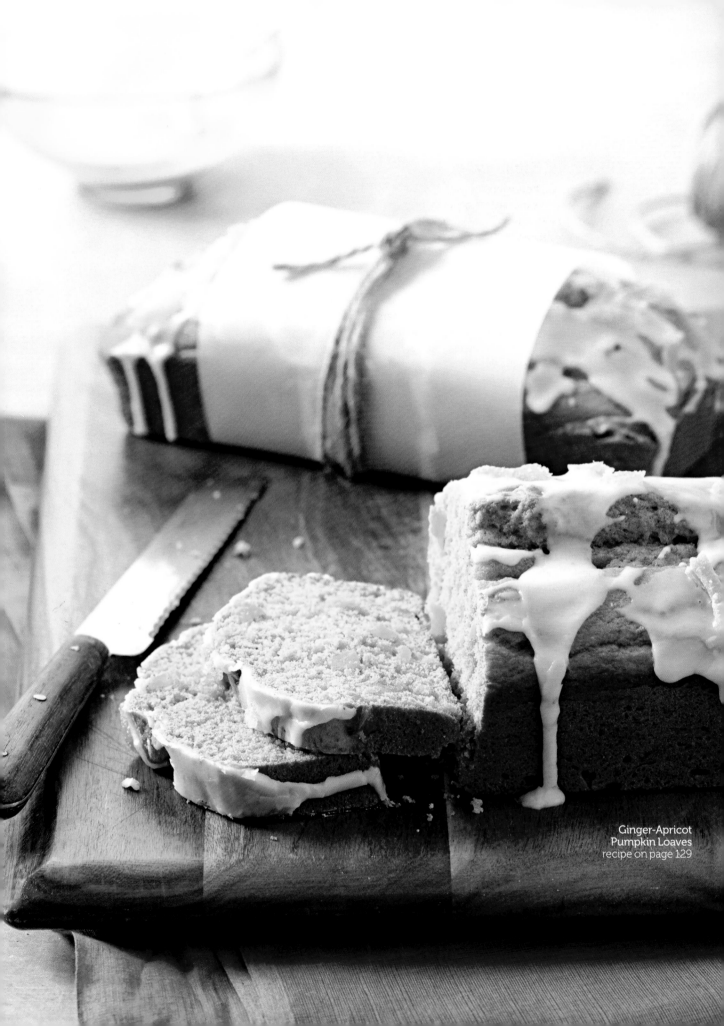

Ginger-Apricot
Pumpkin Loaves
recipe on page 129

Traditions make holiday celebrations special.

Decorating the tree, wrapping gifts, and baking cookies as a family can create memories that last for generations. At our house, just as necessary to holiday tradition is the food we eat. Over the years, I have accumulated a treasury of recipes that I usually reserve for festive meals and other important occasions. Some are specialties that have been passed from one generation to the next. Others are new dishes that have quickly become favorites.

Serving food that is good for my family is as important to me as serving food that tastes good. Through the years, I have found simple ways to adapt treasured family recipes into dishes that are more healthful. That's why I always look forward to the newest issue of *Diabetic Living* magazine as well as the latest volume of *Holiday Cooking*. These publications are full of innovative, new recipe ideas as well as classics that have been updated to ensure great-tasting dishes that are health-smart and easy to prepare.

This year, instead of a traditional breakfast strata, try Squash and Bacon Breakfast Bake, *page 9*. For a new dinnertime showpiece, turn to Roast Beef with Fig-Cranberry Chutney and Horseradish Potatoes, *page 69*. And, because everyone deserves a little holiday indulgence, finish a meal with Molten Chocolate Cakes with Coconut Cream, *page 154*. You can be sure that each of these recipes, along with all the others in this book, has been lightened in calories, fat, and carbohydrate and fits into diabetes meal plans.

I am already counting down the days until the season is in full force and health-savvy holiday cooking will be showcased once again at my house. I hope you are, too.

Enjoy the season!

Martha

Martha Miller Johnson
Editor, *Diabetic Living*® magazine

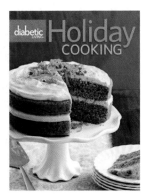

ON THE COVER:

Chai Carrot Cake with Walnuts
recipe on page 144

Photographer: Jason Donnelly

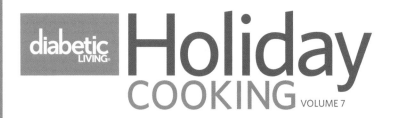

Holiday COOKING VOLUME 7

CONSUMER MARKETING

Vice President, Consumer Marketing	JANET DONNELLY
Consumer Marketing Product Director	HEATHER SORENSEN
Consumer Marketing Product Manager	WENDY MERICAL
Business Director	RON CLINGMAN
Production Manager	AL RODRUCK
Contributing Project Manager	SHELLI McCONNELL, PURPLE PEAR PUBLISHING, INC.
Contributing Photographer	JASON DONNELLY
Contributing Food Stylist	JENNIFER PETERSON
Test Kitchen Director	LYNN BLANCHARD
Test Kitchen Product Supervisors	JANE BURNETT, RD, LD; CARLA CHRISTIAN, RD, LD
Editorial Assistants	LORI EGGERS, MARLENE TODD

SPECIAL INTEREST MEDIA

Editorial Director	JIM BLUME
Senior Design Director	GENE RAUCH
Managing Editor	DOUG KOUMA

DIABETIC LIVING® MAGAZINE

Editor	MARTHA MILLER JOHNSON
Senior Associate Art Director	MICHELLE BILYEU
Senior Associate Editor	JESSIE SHAFER, RD
Assistant Art Director	NIKKI SANDERS

MEREDITH NATIONAL MEDIA GROUP

President **TOM HARTY**

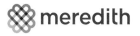

Chairman and Chief Executive Officer **STEPHEN M. LACY**

Vice Chairman **MELL MEREDITH FRAZIER**

In Memoriam — E.T. MEREDITH III (1933-2003)

Diabetic Living® Holiday Cooking is part of a series published by Meredith Corp., 1716 Locust St., Des Moines, IA 50309-3023.

If you have comments or questions about the editorial material in *Diabetic Living® Holiday Cooking*, write to the editor of *Diabetic Living* magazine, Meredith Corp., 1716 Locust St., Des Moines, IA 50309-3023. Send an e-mail to *diabeticlivingmeredith.com* or call 800/678-2651. *Diabetic Living* magazine is available by subscription or on the newsstand. To order a subscription to *Diabetic Living* magazine, go to *DiabeticLivingOnline.com*.

contents

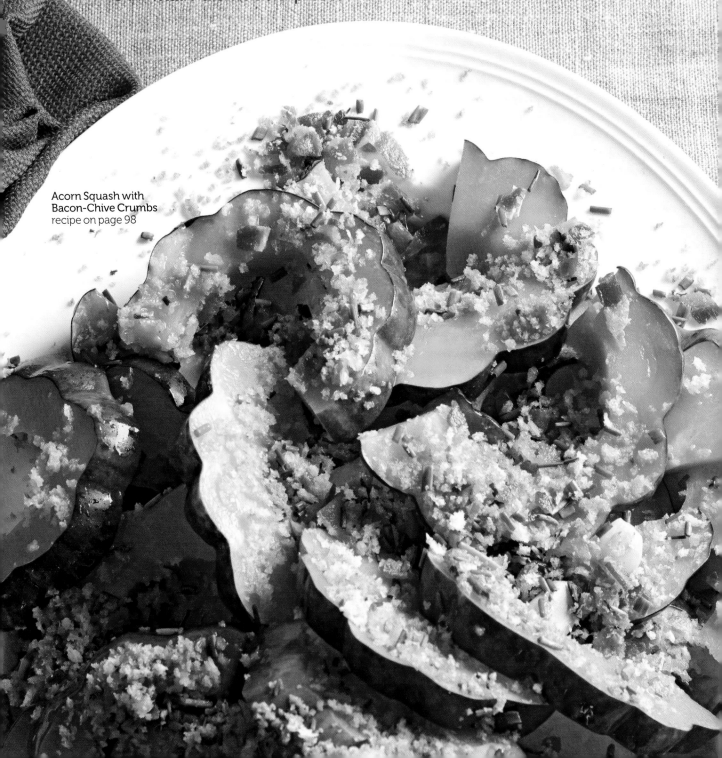

Acorn Squash with Bacon-Chive Crumbs
recipe on page 98

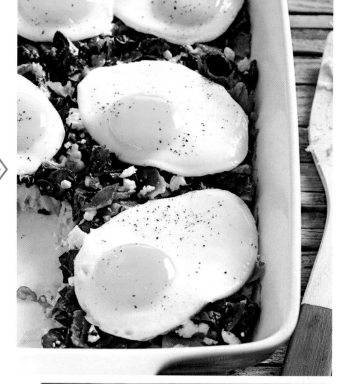

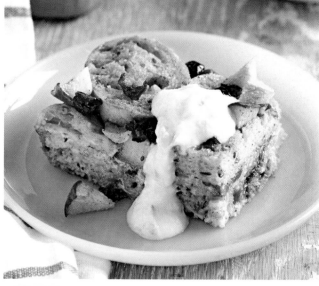

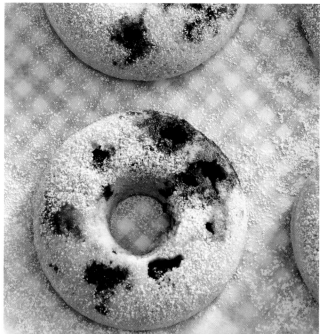

eye-opening
breakfasts

It's refreshing to sit down to breakfast foods that are creatively

new, yet delicious and nutritious. This holiday, dish up one of

these company-special recipes—each is low in calories, fat, and

carbohydrate, making them just right for a diabetes meal plan.

And some of the baked goods are even gluten-free.

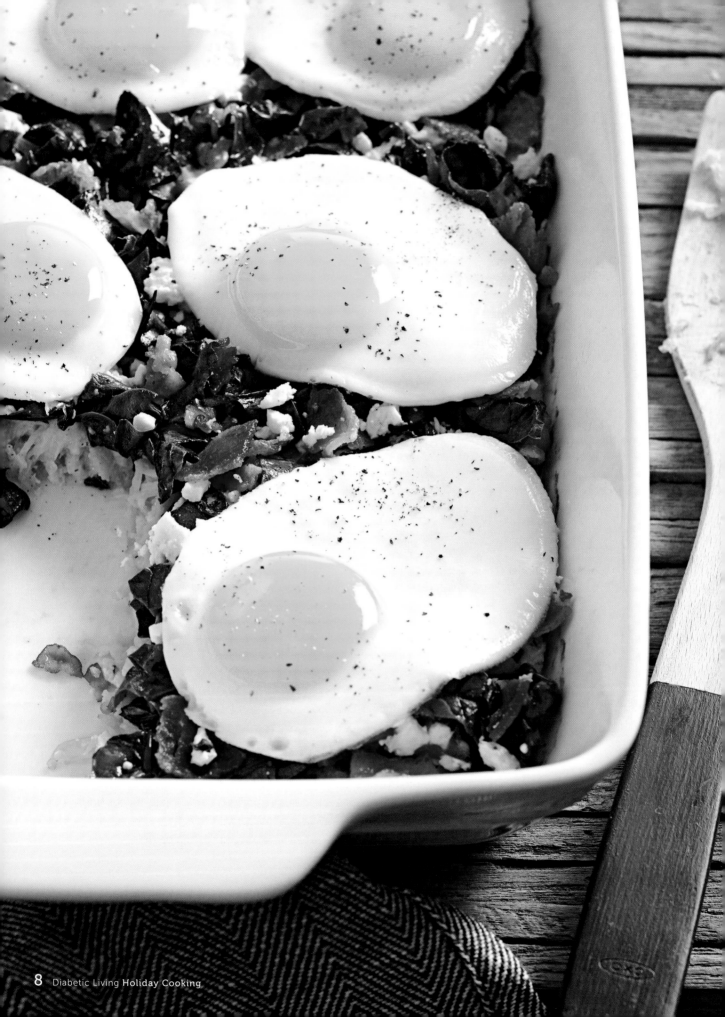

Squash and Bacon Breakfast Bake

Place the eggs on top of the squash bake so each piece will be the same size with an egg centered on top when cut.

SERVINGS 6 ($^1/_6$ of the casserole and 1 egg each)
CARB. PER SERVING 16 g
PREP 35 minutes   COOL 1 hour   BAKE 85 minutes

- 1   3-pound spaghetti squash
- $^1/_2$ cup refrigerated or frozen egg product, thawed, or 2 eggs, lightly beaten
- $^1/_3$ cup finely shredded Parmesan cheese
- 3   tablespoons flour
- 2   tablespoons snipped fresh sage
- 6   slices lower-sodium, less-fat bacon, coarsely chopped

Nonstick cooking spray

- 3   cups coarsely chopped, trimmed Swiss chard
- 2   ounces reduced-fat feta cheese, crumbled (about $^1/_3$ cup)
- 6   eggs
- $^1/_4$ teaspoon salt
- $^1/_4$ teaspoon black pepper

PER SERVING: 213 cal., 10 g total fat (4 g sat. fat), 195 mg chol., 549 mg sodium, 16 g carb. (3 g fiber, 5 g sugars), 16 g pro. Exchanges: 0.5 vegetable, 1 starch, 1.5 medium-fat meat, 0.5 fat.

1 Preheat oven to 375°F. Line a small baking pan with parchment paper. Cut spaghetti squash in half crosswise. Use a spoon to scoop out and discard seeds and strings. Place squash halves, cut sides down, on prepared baking pan. Bake about 1 hour or until squash is tender when pierced with a sharp knife. Cool completely on a wire rack. Reduce oven temperature to 350°F.

2 For crust, in a large bowl combine egg, Parmesan cheese, flour, and sage. Using a fork, scrape squash pulp into the bowl with egg mixture. Gently stir until well combined. Spread mixture evenly in a greased 2-quart rectangular baking dish. Bake, uncovered, about 20 minutes or until crust is set and edges are starting to brown.

3 Meanwhile, in a large nonstick skillet cook bacon over medium heat until just browned but not crisp. Using a slotted spoon, transfer bacon to a small bowl. Discard bacon drippings. Spray skillet with cooking spray. Add chard to skillet; cook and stir for 1 minute.

4 Top squash crust with Swiss chard, feta cheese, and bacon. Bake, uncovered, about 5 minutes more or until heated through.

5 Coat the same skillet with cooking spray. Heat skillet over medium heat. Break three eggs into skillet, keeping eggs separate. Sprinkle with half the salt and half the pepper. Reduce heat to low; cook eggs for 3 to 4 minutes or until whites are completely set and yolks start to thicken. Remove from heat for sunny-side-up eggs. For fried eggs over easy or over hard, when the whites are completely set and yolks start to thicken, turn the eggs and cook for 30 seconds more (for over easy) or 1 minute more (for over hard). Remove eggs from the skillet and position on baked casserole. Repeat with remaining three eggs and remaining salt and pepper.

6 To serve, cut baked casserole into six equal portions and place on six serving plates.

Salmon-Artichoke Omelets

Hot-smoked salmon is usually found in a vacuum-packed package in the meat and seafood area of the supermarket.

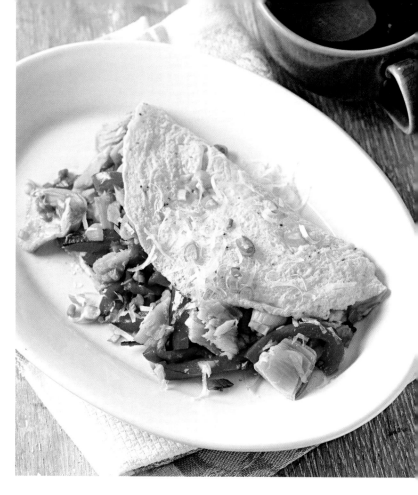

SERVINGS 4 (1 filled omelet each)
CARB. PER SERVING 10 g
PREP 20 minutes   COOK 18 minutes

- 1   large red sweet pepper, cut into thin bite-size strips
- 1   tablespoon olive oil
- 1   14-ounce can quartered artichoke hearts, rinsed, drained, and coarsely chopped
- 2   cloves garlic, minced
- ½   cup sliced green onions (4)
- 2   ounces hot-smoked salmon, skinned, flaked, and bones removed if necessary
- 2   cups refrigerated or frozen egg product, thawed, or 6 eggs and 3 egg whites
- ¼   cup water
- ⅛   teaspoon black pepper
- Nonstick cooking spray
- 4   teaspoons finely shredded Parmesan cheese
- Sliced green onions (optional)

PER SERVING: 150 cal., 5 g total fat (1 g sat. fat), 4 mg chol., 560 mg sodium, 10 g carb. (2 g fiber, 4 g sugars), 16 g pro. Exchanges: 1.5 vegetable, 2 lean meat, 0.5 fat.

1 For filling, in a large skillet cook sweet pepper in hot oil over medium heat about 5 minutes or until just tender, stirring occasionally. Add artichokes and garlic; cook and stir for 30 seconds more. Remove from heat. Stir in the ½ cup green onions and the salmon; set filling aside.

2 In a medium bowl combine egg, water, and black pepper. Using a fork, beat until combined but not frothy. Generously coat a medium nonstick skillet with flared sides with cooking spray; heat over medium-high heat until skillet is hot.

3 Add one-fourth of the egg mixture to skillet; reduce heat to medium. Immediately begin stirring the eggs gently but continuously with a wooden spoon or heatproof spatula until mixture resembles small pieces of cooked egg surrounded by liquid egg. Stop stirring. Cook for 30 to 60 seconds more or until egg is set and shiny.

4 Spoon one-fourth of the filling mixture (about ¾ cup) across one side of the omelet. With a spatula lift the opposite side of egg over filling. Transfer omelet to a serving plate; sprinkle with 1 teaspoon of the Parmesan cheese. Cover with foil to keep warm. Repeat with remaining egg mixture and filling mixture to make three more omelets. If desired, sprinkle with additional sliced green onions. Serve immediately.

Spanish Eggs

Instead of toast, serve this spicy breakfast dish with warmed yellow or white corn tortillas.

SERVINGS 4 (1 egg and 1 cup tomato mixture each)
CARB. PER SERVING 12 g
START TO FINISH 30 minutes

½ cup chopped onion (1 medium)

1 small fresh Anaheim chile pepper, stemmed, seeded, and chopped*

1 clove garlic, minced

1 tablespoon olive oil

2 14.5-ounce cans no-salt-added fire-roasted diced tomatoes, undrained

1 small zucchini, halved lengthwise and thinly sliced (1¼ cups)

½ teaspoon salt

2 tablespoons snipped fresh cilantro

4 eggs

Crumbled queso fresco (optional)

Fresh cilantro sprigs (optional)

1 | In a large skillet cook onion, chile pepper, and garlic in hot oil over medium heat about 5 minutes or until tender. Add tomatoes, zucchini, and salt; cook 5 minutes more or until zucchini is just tender. Stir in snipped cilantro.

2 | Break one of the eggs into a measuring cup. Carefully slide egg into the tomato mixture. Repeat with the remaining three eggs, allowing each egg an equal amount of space in the tomato mixture. Cover and simmer over medium-low heat for 3 to 5 minutes or until whites are completely set and yolks begin to thicken but are not hard. If desired, sprinkle with queso fresco and garnish with fresh cilantro sprigs.

*TEST KITCHEN TIP: Because chile peppers contain volatile oils that can burn your skin and eyes, avoid direct contact with them as much as possible. When working with chile peppers, wear plastic or rubber gloves. If your bare hands do touch the peppers, wash your hands and nails with soap and warm water.

QUICK TIP
To easily snip fresh herbs, place the herb leaves in a glass measuring cup. Use kitchen scissors to snip the herbs into pieces.

PER SERVING: 168 cal., 8 g total fat (2 g sat. fat), 186 mg chol., 390 mg sodium, 12 g carb. (3 g fiber, 7 g sugars), 9 g pro. Exchanges: 2 vegetable, 1 medium-fat meat, 0.5 fat.

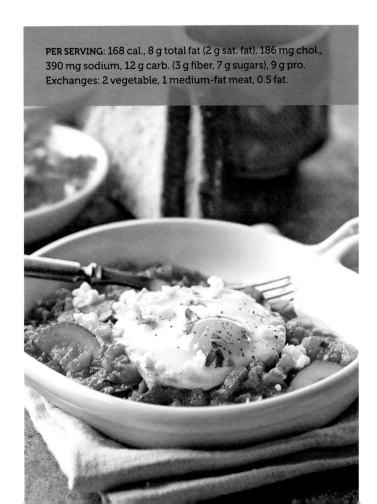

Feta-Kale Quiches with Warm Tomato Jam

Kale can be purchased in a bunch or washed and torn in a bag. If you purchase a bunch, tear the green leafy parts from the stem and use a chef's knife to chop the leaves.

SERVINGS 6 (1 quiche and 1$\frac{1}{2}$ tablespoons tomato jam each)
CARB. PER SERVING 13 g
PREP 25 minutes   COOK 13 minutes
BAKE 20 minutes

- 4 sheets frozen phyllo dough (14×9-inch rectangles), thawed

  Butter-flavor nonstick cooking spray

- 1$\frac{1}{2}$ cups chopped fresh kale
- 2 tablespoons water
- 1$\frac{3}{4}$ cups refrigerated or frozen egg product, thawed, or 7 eggs, lightly beaten
- $\frac{1}{4}$ cup crumbled reduced-fat feta cheese
- 2 to 3 tablespoons finely chopped, rinsed and drained jarred sweet piquante peppers*
- 2 teaspoons snipped fresh rosemary or fresh thyme
- $\frac{1}{2}$ cup chopped onion
- 1 teaspoon butter
- 1 cup chopped fresh tomatoes, or $\frac{3}{4}$ cup canned no-salt-added diced tomatoes, drained
- 1 tablespoon packed brown sugar**
- 1 tablespoon red wine vinegar
- $\frac{1}{8}$ teaspoon salt

PER SERVING: 108 cal., 2 g total fat (1 g sat. fat), 3 mg chol., 310 mg sodium, 13 g carb. (1 g fiber, 5 g sugars), 10 g pro. Exchanges: 1 vegetable, 0.5 starch, 1 lean meat.

1 Preheat oven to 350°F. Unfold phyllo dough; remove one sheet and lay on a clean flat surface. (As you work, cover remaining phyllo dough with plastic wrap to prevent it from drying out.) Lightly coat phyllo sheet with cooking spray. Top with a second phyllo sheet; coat again with cooking spray. Cut the stack into six rectangles by cutting in half lengthwise and then in thirds crosswise. Repeat with remaining two sheets of phyllo to make a second stack. Cut the second stack into six rectangles as directed above.

2 Lay one phyllo rectangle in each of six 6-ounce custard cups, pressing the phyllo rectangle down into the cup so it is pressed onto the bottom and up the sides. Lay the remaining phyllo rectangles across the first rectangles in the cups and press down into the cups so that the cup is completely lined with phyllo. Set cups in a 15×10×1-inch baking pan; set aside.

3 In a medium skillet cook kale and water, covered, over medium heat for 1 minute. Uncover and cook for 2 to 4 minutes more or until kale is nearly tender and water is evaporated. In a medium bowl combine egg, feta cheese, peppers, and rosemary. Stir in kale. Spoon egg mixture evenly into phyllo-lined custard cups.

4 Bake quiches for 20 to 25 minutes or until a knife inserted in centers comes out clean.

5 Meanwhile, for tomato jam, in a medium skillet cook onion in hot butter over medium heat about 5 minutes or until tender, stirring occasionally. Add tomatoes. Cook for 3 to 5 minutes more or until tomatoes are tender, stirring occasionally and mashing tomatoes with a fork or potato masher. Add brown sugar, vinegar, and salt. Continue to cook for 2 to 3 minutes more or until jam is slightly thickened.

6 Let quiches cool in cups on a wire rack for 5 minutes. Carefully lift quiches from cups and place one on each of six plates. Spoon warm tomato jam over quiches to serve.

*TEST KITCHEN TIP: If desired, substitute chopped jarred roasted red sweet peppers for the piquante peppers.

**SUGAR SUBSTITUTE: We do not recommend using a sugar substitute for this recipe.

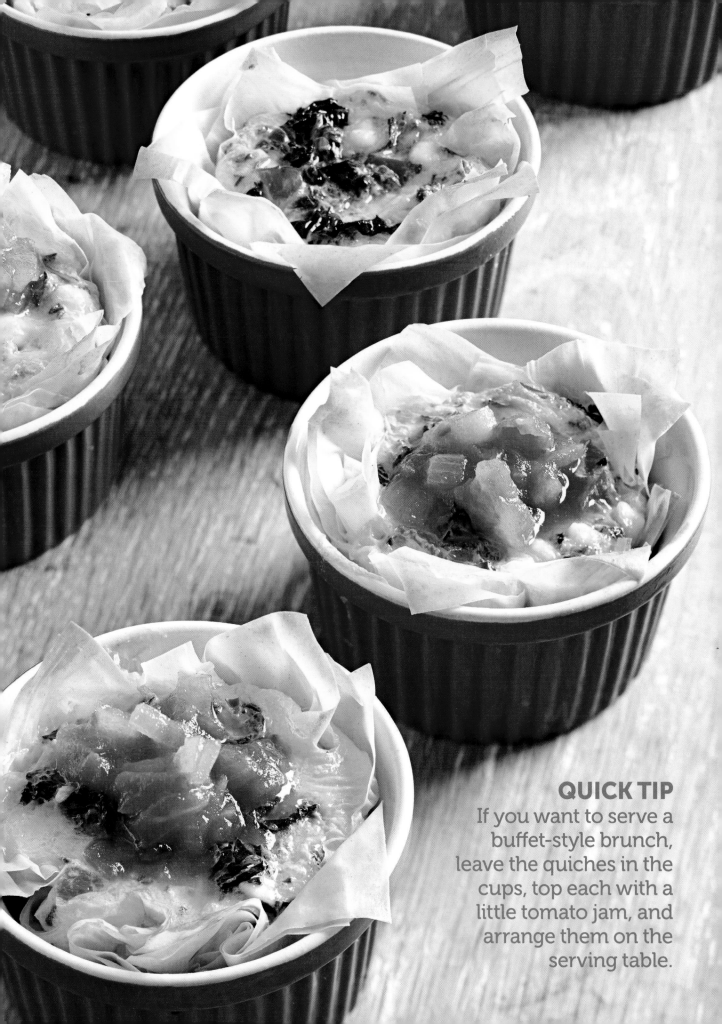

QUICK TIP
If you want to serve a buffet-style brunch, leave the quiches in the cups, top each with a little tomato jam, and arrange them on the serving table.

Crab Cake Egg Stacks

Look for mango chutney along with other condiments in the supermarket. If it has large pieces of fruit, snip them with kitchen scissors.

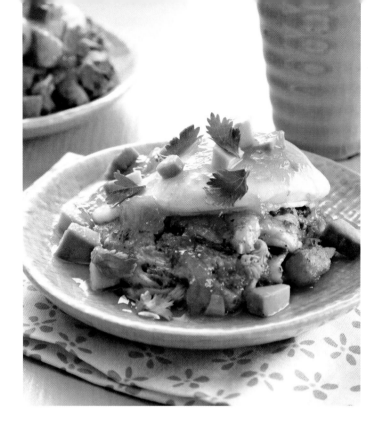

SERVINGS 5 (1 crab cake, 1 egg, and about 2^1/$_2$ tablespoons topper each)
CARB. PER SERVING 12 g
PREP 30 minutes   COOK 10 minutes

- 1 6-ounce pouch refrigerated lump crabmeat, rinsed, drained, and flaked
- 1 cup shredded zucchini
- 2 egg whites
- 2 tablespoons plain fat-free Greek yogurt
- 3 tablespoons whole wheat panko bread crumbs
- ^{1}/$_2$ teaspoon chili powder
- ^{1}/$_4$ teaspoon black pepper
- ^{1}/$_4$ teaspoon crushed red pepper
- Nonstick cooking spray
- 2 tablespoons mango chutney
- 1 avocado, halved, seeded, peeled, and chopped
- 1 teaspoon lemon juice
- 5 eggs, poached*
- Bottled hot pepper sauce
- ^{1}/$_4$ cup snipped fresh cilantro (optional)

PER SERVING: 193 cal., 9 g total fat (2 g sat. fat), 231 mg chol., 310 mg sodium, 12 g carb. (2 g fiber, 5 g sugars), 16 g pro. Exchanges: 1 fruit, 2 lean meat, 1 fat.

1 | In a medium bowl combine crabmeat, zucchini, egg whites, and yogurt. Stir in panko, chili powder, black pepper, and crushed red pepper.

2 | Form mixture into five ^{1}/$_2$-inch-thick patties (about ^{1}/$_3$ cup crab mixture per patty). Coat a large nonstick skillet with cooking spray. Heat skillet over medium-high heat. Add patties to hot skillet; cook about 10 minutes or until lightly browned (160°F), turning once halfway through cooking time. Reduce heat as needed to prevent the patties from overbrowning.

3 | Meanwhile, for avocado topper, snip any large pieces of chutney. In a small bowl stir together chutney, avocado, and lemon juice.

4 | Serve each crab cake topped with a poached egg. Spoon avocado topper over all. Sprinkle each serving with 1 or 2 dashes of hot pepper sauce. If desired, garnish with snipped cilantro.

*TEST KITCHEN TIP: To poach eggs, fill an extra-large skillet half full of water; add 1 tablespoon vinegar. Bring the vinegar mixture to boiling; reduce heat to simmering. Break 1 egg into a cup and slip egg into the simmering water. Repeat with four more eggs, allowing each egg an equal amount of space in the vinegar mixture. Simmer eggs, uncovered, for 3 to 5 minutes or until whites are completely set and yolks begin to thicken but are not hard. Using a slotted spoon, remove eggs from vinegar mixture.

Asparagus, Prosciutto, and Arugula Breakfast Sandwiches

Select asparagus spears that are similar in size—this will guarantee even cooking.

SERVINGS 4 (1 sandwich each)
CARB. PER SERVING 31 g
START TO FINISH 20 minutes

12 asparagus spears, trimmed and halved crosswise

Nonstick cooking spray

4 eggs

4 Cheddar Biscuits (see recipe, *page 135*)

1 cup baby arugula

4 very thin slices prosciutto

6 teaspoons pure maple syrup

Black pepper (optional)

1 In a covered large saucepan cook asparagus in a small amount of boiling water for 5 to 8 minutes or just until tender. Drain.

2 Meanwhile, coat a large nonstick skillet with cooking spray. Heat skillet over medium heat. Break eggs into skillet, keeping eggs separate. Reduce heat to low; cook eggs for 3 to 4 minutes or until whites are completely set and yolks start to thicken. For fried eggs over hard, turn the eggs and cook about 1 minute more or until desired doneness.

3 Split each Cheddar Biscuit. Arrange arugula on bottoms of biscuits. Top with prosciutto. Drizzle with maple syrup. Top each sandwich with one-fourth of the cooked asparagus and one egg. If desired, sprinkle with pepper. Add biscuit tops.

PER SERVING: 285 cal., 11 g total fat (4 g sat. fat), 203 mg chol., 575 mg sodium, 31 g carb. (2 g fiber, 8 g sugars), 15 g pro. Exchanges: 1.5 starch, 0.5 carb., 1.5 medium-fat meat, 1 fat.

11 grams fat

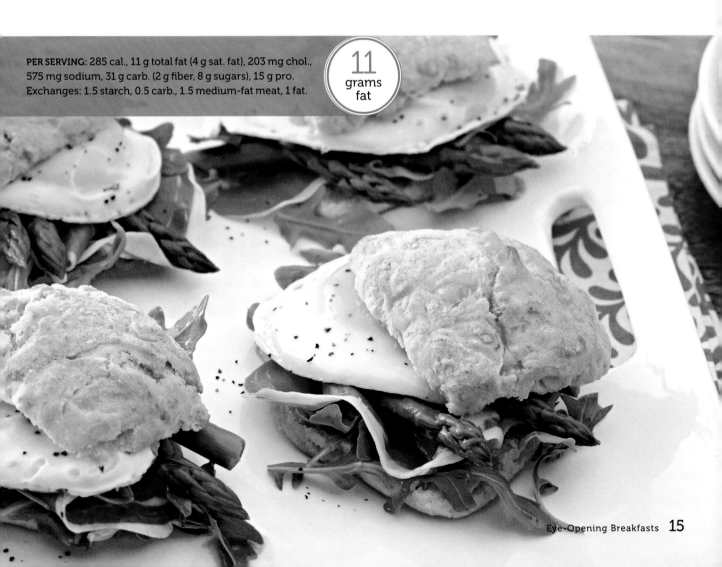

Asparagus, Zucchini, and Yellow Pepper Frittata

Shredded mozzarella or provolone cheese can be substitued for the mild, nutty Fontina cheese that's sprinkled on top of this Italian-style egg casserole.

SERVINGS 8 (1 portion each)
CARB. PER SERVING 9 g
PREP 30 minutes **BAKE** 35 minutes
STAND 10 minutes

1½ pounds fresh asparagus or two 9- or 10-ounce packages frozen cut asparagus

1 medium yellow sweet pepper, cut into ¼-inch-wide strips

⅓ cup chopped onion (1 small)

1 small zucchini, halved lengthwise and cut into ¼-inch-thick slices (about 1 cup)

4½ cups refrigerated or frozen egg product, thawed, or 10 eggs, lightly beaten

1 cup low-fat milk

2 tablespoons snipped fresh Italian (flat-leaf) parsley

¾ teaspoon salt

¼ to ½ teaspoon black pepper

2 ounces Fontina cheese, shredded (½ cup)

PER SERVING: 131 cal., 3 g total fat (2 g sat. fat), 10 mg chol., 551 mg sodium, 9 g carb. (2 g fiber, 5 g sugars), 18 g pro. Exchanges: 1 vegetable, 2 lean meat.

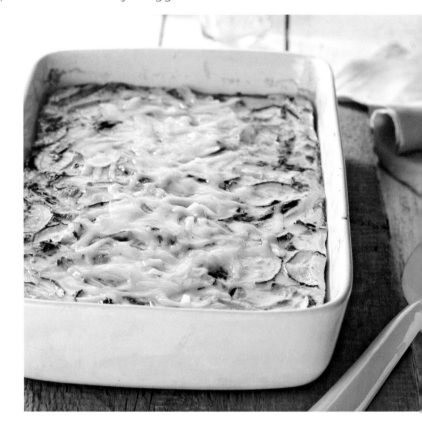

1 Preheat oven to 350°F. Grease a 2-quart rectangular baking dish; set aside.

2 If using fresh asparagus, snap off and discard woody bases. Cut fresh asparagus into 1-inch pieces.

3 In a large saucepan bring about 1 inch water to boiling. Add asparagus, sweet pepper strips, and onion. Return just to boiling; reduce heat slightly. Boil, covered, about 1 minute or until crisp-tender. Drain well. Spread the asparagus-pepper mixture evenly in prepared baking dish. Layer with zucchini slices.

4 In a large bowl combine egg, milk, parsley, salt, and black pepper. Pour over vegetables in baking dish. Sprinkle with cheese. Bake, uncovered, about 35 minutes or until a knife inserted near the center comes out clean. Let stand for 10 minutes before cutting into eight portions.

Breakfast "Risotto" with Fried Eggs

Risotto is a creamy rice dish common in Italian cuisine. Steel-cut oats take the place of Arborio rice in this hearty breakfast dish.

SERVINGS 8 (1 egg with $1/2$ cup oatmeal mixture each)
CARB. PER SERVING 16 g
PREP 10 minutes COOK 30 minutes

Nonstick cooking spray

$3/4$ cup chopped red sweet pepper (1 medium)

1 cup sliced fresh button or cremini mushrooms

3 tablespoons thinly sliced green onions

3 cups water

$1/4$ teaspoon salt

1 cup steel-cut oats

2 ounces reduced-fat or light Brie cheese, rind removed

1 ounce reduced-fat cream cheese (Neufchâtel), softened

2 cups coarsely chopped fresh spinach

8 eggs

$1/4$ cup snipped fresh basil

Freshly ground black pepper

1 | Coat a large nonstick saucepan with cooking spray; heat over medium heat. Add sweet pepper and mushrooms. Cook for 5 minutes, stirring occasionally. Add green onions and cook for 3 minutes more, stirring occasionally. Remove vegetables from saucepan; set aside.

2 | In a medium saucepan bring the water and salt to boiling; reduce heat to low and cover. Add oats to the saucepan used to cook the vegetables.

3 | Carefully stir 1 cup of the simmering water into the oats. Cook, stirring frequently, over medium heat until liquid is absorbed. Stir another 1 cup of the water into the oats. Continue to cook, stirring frequently, until liquid is absorbed. Stir $1/2$ cup of the water into oat mixture. Cook, stirring frequently, until water is absorbed. Stir in the remaining water. Cook and stir until oats are just tender.

4 | Remove oat mixture from the heat. Add Brie cheese and cream cheese. Stir until cheese is melted and mixture is well combined. Stir in spinach and reserved vegetable mixture.

5 | Meanwhile, coat a large nonstick skillet with cooking spray. Heat skillet over medium heat. Break eggs into skillet, keeping eggs separate. Reduce heat to low; cook eggs for 3 to 4 minutes or until whites are completely set and yolks start to thicken. For fried eggs over easy or over hard, turn the eggs and cook for 30 seconds more (for over easy) or 1 minute more (for over hard).

6 | To serve, spoon oat mixture into four shallow bowls. Top each serving with an egg, yolk side up. Sprinkle with basil and freshly ground black pepper.

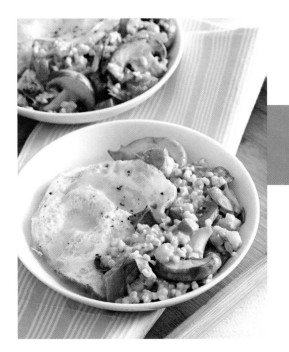

PER SERVING: 183 cal., 8 g total fat (3 g sat. fat), 192 mg chol., 223 mg sodium, 16 g carb. (3 g fiber, 2 g sugars), 12 g pro. Exchanges: 1 starch, 1 medium-fat meat, 0.5 fat.

16 grams carb.

Pear-Cranberry French Toast with Orange-Ricotta Cream

Try dried tart red cherries, dried blueberries, or golden raisins in place of the dried cranberries.

SERVINGS 12 (1 portion French toast and 2 tablespoons ricotta cream each)
CARB. PER SERVING 28 g
PREP 45 minutes BAKE 35 minutes STAND 10 minutes

2 7-ounce loaves whole grain baguette-style bread

1 medium fresh red pear, cored and chopped

½ cup dried cranberries, snipped

5 eggs

1¼ cups fat-free milk

3 tablespoons reduced-calorie maple-flavor syrup

1 tablespoon packed brown sugar*

1 teaspoon pumpkin pie spice

1 teaspoon vanilla

¼ teaspoon salt

1 6-ounce carton plain fat-free or low-fat Greek yogurt

½ cup light ricotta cheese

2 tablespoons honey

1 tablespoon very finely chopped crystallized ginger

1 teaspoon finely shredded orange peel

1 Preheat oven to 350°F. Grease a 2-quart rectangular baking dish; set aside. Trim rounded ends off baguettes and discard. Cut baguettes crosswise into ½-inch slices. To assemble, arrange half of the bread slices in the bottom of the prepared baking dish. Top with half the pears and half the cranberries. Repeat layers.

2 In a medium bowl whisk together eggs, milk, maple-flavor syrup, brown sugar, pumpkin pie spice, vanilla, and salt. Slowly pour egg mixture evenly over bread slices.**

3 Bake, uncovered, for 35 to 40 minutes or until a knife inserted in center comes out clean. Let stand for 10 minutes before serving.

4 While the French toast bakes, prepare the ricotta cream. In a small bowl combine yogurt, ricotta cheese, honey, ginger, and orange peel. Set aside.

5 To serve, cut French toast into twelve portions. Divide among twelve serving plates. Spoon ricotta cream evenly over French toast. Serve warm.

*SUGAR SUBSTITUTE: We do not recommend using a sugar substitute for this recipe.

**MAKE-AHEAD DIRECTIONS: Do not preheat oven in Step 1. Prepare according to directions through Step 2. Cover and chill for 2 to 24 hours. Preheat oven to 350°F. Continue with Step 3 as directed.

4 grams fat

PER SERVING: 177 cal., 4 g total fat (1 g sat. fat), 81 mg chol., 236 mg sodium, 28 g carb. (2 g fiber, 14 g sugars), 8 g pro. Exchanges: 1 starch, 1 carb., 1 medium-fat meat.

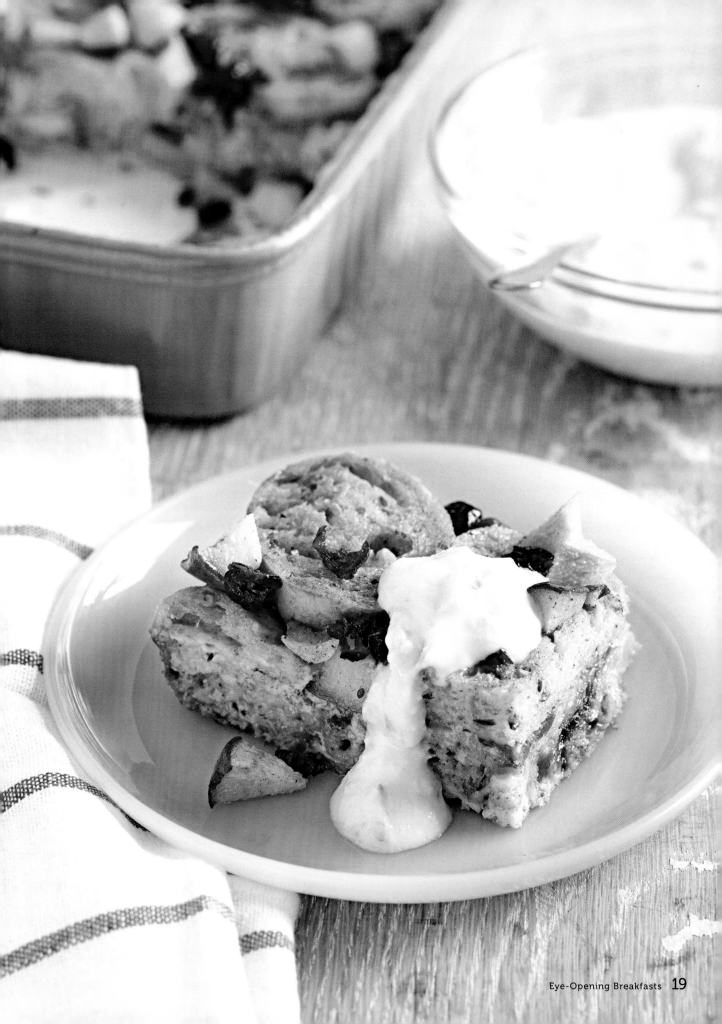

Chai Breakfast Muffins

The subtle spiced-tea flavor comes through in each bite of these cakey muffins.

SERVINGS 24 (1 muffin each)
CARB. PER SERVING 24 g
PREP 25 minutes BAKE 15 minutes
COOL 5 minutes

Nonstick cooking spray

1½ cups all-purpose flour

½ cup whole wheat flour

1½ teaspoons baking powder

½ teaspoon baking soda

½ teaspoon ground ginger

¼ teaspoon salt

1 cup fat-free milk

4 chai tea bags

½ cup butter, softened

1½ cups sugar*

½ teaspoon vanilla

½ cup refrigerated or frozen egg product, thawed, or 2 eggs

¾ cup maple-flavor granola or granola with dried fruit

1 | Preheat oven to 350°F. Line twenty-four 2½-inch muffin cups with paper bake cups. Lightly coat bake cups with cooking spray; set aside. In a medium bowl stir together all-purpose flour, whole wheat flour, baking powder, baking soda, ginger, and salt. In a small saucepan heat milk just until simmering. Remove from heat. Add tea bags; steep for 5 minutes. Remove tea bags, pressing bags to release excess tea back into saucepan. Cool.

2 | In a large mixing bowl beat butter with an electric mixer on medium to high speed about 1 minute or until fluffy. Add sugar and vanilla; beat until combined. Add egg, half at a time, beating well after each addition. Alternately add flour mixture and milk mixture to butter mixture, beating on low speed after each addition just until combined.

3 | Spoon batter into prepared muffin cups, filling each about two-thirds full. Sprinkle with granola.

4 | Bake for 15 to 20 minutes or until a wooden toothpick inserted in centers comes out clean. Cool in muffin cups on wire racks for 5 minutes. Remove muffins from cups. Serve warm.

*SUGAR SUBSTITUTE: We do not recommend using a sugar substitute for this recipe.

PER SERVING: 143 cal., 5 g total fat (2 g sat. fat), 10 mg chol., 132 mg sodium, 24 g carb. (1 g fiber, 14 g sugars), 3 g pro. Exchanges: 0.5 starch, 1 carb., 1 fat.

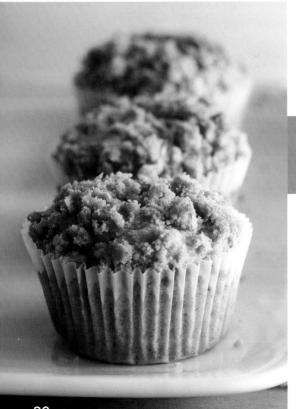

Gluten-Free Pumpkin Waffles

Because you use only a little of each specialty flour, store the remaining in freezer containers or bags and freeze for up to 6 months.

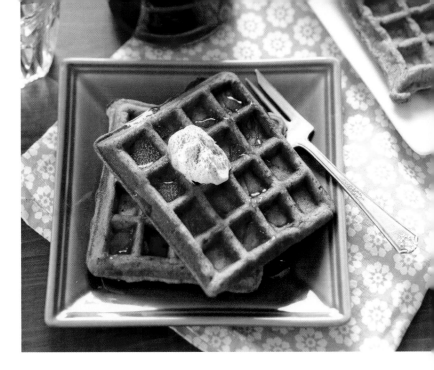

SERVINGS 6 (2 4-inch square waffles [$^1/_4$ cup batter per waffle] each)
CARB. PER SERVING 26 g or 21 g
PREP 20 minutes **STAND** 5 minutes
BAKE per waffle baker directions

Nonstick cooking spray

$^1/_2$ cup gluten-free all-purpose flour

$^1/_2$ cup vanilla-flavor whey protein powder

$^1/_4$ cup coconut flour

$^1/_4$ cup flaxseed meal

$^1/_4$ cup sugar*

2 teaspoons arrowroot or cornstarch

2 teaspoons baking powder

2 teaspoons ground cinnamon

$^1/_2$ teaspoon baking soda

$^1/_2$ teaspoon ground ginger

1 cup unsweetened almond milk

$^3/_4$ cup canned pumpkin**

3 egg whites

1 tablespoon grapeseed oil

1 teaspoon vanilla

Sugar-free maple syrup (optional)

Frozen light whipped dessert topping, thawed (optional)

Ground cinnamon (optional)

PER SERVING: 196 cal., 6 g total fat (1 g sat. fat), 23 mg chol., 338 mg sodium, 26 g carb. (6 g fiber, 10 g sugars), 13 g pro. Exchanges: 0.5 vegetable, 1 starch, 0.5 carb., 1.5 lean meat, 1 fat.

PER SERVING WITH SUBSTITUTE: Same as above, except 183 cal., 21 g carb. (6 g sugars). Exchanges: 0 carb.

1 Lightly coat waffle baker with cooking spray. Preheat a waffle baker on high (the waffle baker needs to be well heated to avoid sticking). Preheat oven to 200°F. Set a wire rack on a baking sheet; place in oven while it's preheating.

2 Meanwhile, in a medium bowl combine gluten-free all-purpose flour, whey protein powder, coconut flour, flaxseed meal, sugar, arrowroot, baking powder, the 2 teaspoons cinnamon, the baking soda, and ginger.

3 In a large bowl whisk together almond milk, pumpkin, egg whites, grapeseed oil, and vanilla. Add flour mixture to pumpkin mixture; stir until well mixed. Let stand for 5 to 10 minutes or until batter thickens.

4 Spoon a scant $^1/_4$ cup of the batter into each section of the waffle baker; spread batter to cover grids. Close lid quickly; do not open until done. Bake according to manufacturer's directions. When done, use a fork to lift waffle off grid; transfer waffle to wire rack in oven. Repeat with the remaining batter. Serve warm. If desired, serve with syrup, dessert topping, and/or additional cinnamon.

*SUGAR SUBSTITUTES: Choose from Splenda Sugar Blend, C&H Light Sugar Blend, or Truvia Sugar Blend. Follow package directions to use product amount equivalent to $^1/_4$ cup sugar.

**TEST KITCHEN TIP: For best results, use a thick canned pumpkin such as Whole Foods 365 Everyday Value brand. If needed to remove excess moisture, spread the pumpkin puree onto a few layers of paper towels; top with several more paper towels and press gently.

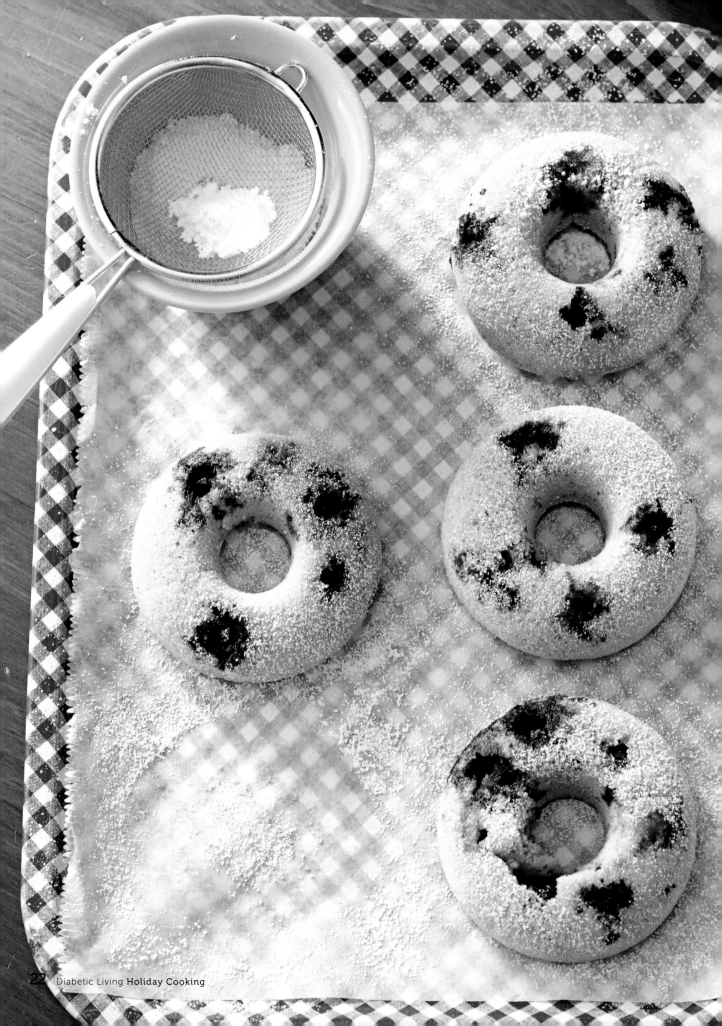

Gluten-Free Blueberry-Lemon Doughnuts

Doughnut pans are typically designed with six molded cups. Because recipes sometimes make more than six doughnuts, it's handy to have more than one pan.

SERVINGS 9 (1 doughnut each)
CARB. PER SERVING 19 g or 16 g
PREP 25 minutes   BAKE 15 minutes   COOL 5 minutes

2 teaspoons canola oil

2 teaspoons gluten-free all-purpose flour

½ cup almond flour

½ cup gluten-free oat flour

½ cup gluten-free all-purpose flour

¼ cup granulated sugar*

2 tablespoons vanilla-flavor whey protein powder

1½ teaspoons baking powder

¼ teaspoon baking soda

¼ teaspoon salt

¼ cup plain low-fat yogurt

¼ cup unsweetened almond milk

2 eggs

1 tablespoon finely shredded lemon peel

1 tablespoon canola oil

½ teaspoon vanilla

54 fresh blueberries (½ cup)

1 teaspoon powdered sugar*

PER SERVING: 164 cal., 8 g total fat (1 g sat. fat), 43 mg chol., 208 mg sodium, 19 g carb. (2 g fiber, 8 g sugars), 6 g pro. Exchanges: 1 starch, 0.5 carb., 1.5 fat.

PER SERVING WITH SUBSTITUTE: Same as above, except 156 cal., 16 g carb. (5 g sugars). Exchanges: 0 carb.

1 Preheat oven to 325°F. In a small bowl stir together the 2 teaspoons canola oil and the 2 teaspoons gluten-free all-purpose flour. Coat the six cups of a 3½-inch doughnut pan with some of the oil-flour mixture; set aside.

2 In a medium bowl stir together the almond flour, gluten-free oat flour, the ½ cup gluten-free all-purpose flour, the granulated sugar, whey protein powder, baking powder, baking soda, and salt.

3 In a large bowl whisk together yogurt, almond milk, eggs, lemon peel, the 1 tablespoon oil, and the vanilla until well mixed.

4 Add the flour mixture to the yogurt mixture; whisk until well mixed.

5 Spoon two-thirds of the mixture into prepared cups in doughnut pan, using about ¼ cup of the batter for each cup; spread batter evenly. Arrange six blueberries** in the batter for each doughnut. Bake about 15 minutes or until doughnuts spring back when lightly touched. Cool in pan on a wire rack for 5 minutes. Using a thin metal spatula or table knife, loosen edges of doughnuts. Invert pan and tap on counter to release the doughnuts.

6 Thoroughly wash and dry the doughnut pan. Coat three of the cups with the remaining oil-flour mixture. Fill these cups with the remaining batter and the remaining blueberries. Bake, cool, and remove as directed in Step 5. Serve warm or cool. Before serving, sift powdered sugar over doughnuts.

*SUGAR SUBSTITUTES: For the granulated sugar, choose from Splenda Sugar Blend, C&H Light, or Truvia Baking Blend. Follow package directions to use product amount equivalent to ¼ cup granulated sugar. We do not recommend using a sugar substitute for the powdered sugar.

**TEST KITCHEN TIP: Placing blueberries evenly in the cups helps to prevent the doughnuts from sticking in the cups.

Gluten-Free Strawberry Breakfast Bars

These fruity bars are great for toting for treat day at the office. The bright red fruit filling makes a pretty holiday presentation.

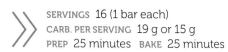

SERVINGS 16 (1 bar each)
CARB. PER SERVING 19 g or 15 g
PREP 25 minutes **BAKE** 25 minutes

Nonstick cooking spray

3 cups chopped fresh strawberries

¼ cup sugar*

4 tablespoons water

1 tablespoon arrowroot

1 cup gluten-free oat flour

1 cup flaxseed meal

½ cup gluten-free all-purpose flour

¼ cup sugar*

1½ teaspoons baking powder

½ teaspoon salt

½ teaspoon xanthan gum

½ teaspoon ground cinnamon

5 tablespoons butter, melted

1 teaspoon vanilla

¼ cup water

1 Preheat oven to 375°F. Lightly coat a 9×9×2-inch baking pan with cooking spray; set aside. For filling, in a medium saucepan combine strawberries, ¼ cup sugar, and 2 tablespoons of the water. Bring to boiling; reduce heat. Simmer, uncovered, about 5 minutes or until strawberries are softened. Using the back of a fork or a potato masher, partially mash berries in saucepan.

2 In a small bowl whisk together the remaining 2 tablespoons water and the arrowroot; stir into the simmering berry mixture. Pour berry mixture into a medium bowl; let cool.

3 For crust, in another medium bowl whisk together gluten-free oat flour, flaxseed meal, gluten-free all-purpose flour, ¼ cup sugar, the baking powder, salt, xanthan gum powder, and cinnamon. Add melted butter and vanilla; toss to combine. Stir in the ¼ cup water; toss until mixture forms a dough.

4 Using your fingers, press two-thirds of the crust firmly and evenly into the prepared baking pan. Spoon filling over top, spreading evenly. Crumble the remaining one-third of the crust over the filling; press gently to adhere.

5 Bake for 25 minutes. Let cool in pan on a wire rack. Cut into 16 bars. Store in the refrigerator for up to 5 days.

*SUGAR SUBSTITUTES: Choose from Splenda Sugar Blend, C&H Light, or Truvia Baking Blend. Follow package directions to use product amounts equivalent to ¼ cup sugar for the filling and ¼ cup sugar for the crust.

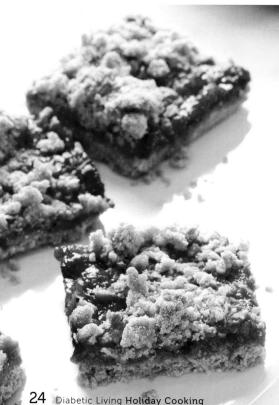

PER SERVING: 141 cal., 7 g total fat (2 g sat. fat), 10 mg chol., 152 mg sodium, 19 g carb. (4 g fiber, 8 g sugars), 3 g pro. Exchanges: 0.5 fruit, 0.5 starch, 1.5 fat.

PER SERVING WITH SUBSTITUTE: Same as above, except 131 cal., 15 g carb. (4 g sugars).

Gluten-Free Cinnamon Crunch Cereal

The cereal bakes in crackerlike sheets that are easy to break into bite-size pieces. Cool the cereal completely before breaking.

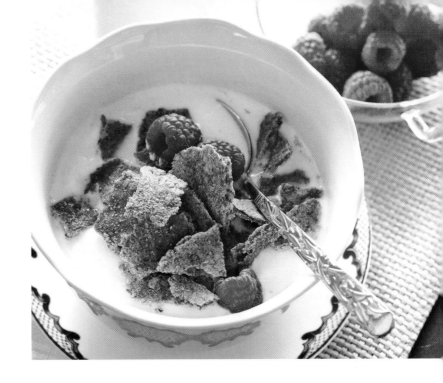

SERVINGS 6 (²/₃ cup each)
CARB. PER SERVING 30 g or 26 g
PREP 25 minutes BAKE 30 minutes
COOL 2 hours 30 minutes

- ¾ cup gluten-free all-purpose flour
- ¾ cup gluten-free oat flour
- ½ cup flaxseed meal
- ⅓ cup almond flour
- 1 teaspoon ground cinnamon
- ½ teaspoon salt
- ½ cup water
- ½ teaspoon vanilla
- ½ teaspoon liquid stevia sweetener (optional)
- 2 tablespoons sugar*
- ½ teaspoon ground cinnamon
- Fat-free milk (optional)
- Fresh berries (optional)

PER SERVING: 205 cal., 8 g total fat (0 g sat. fat), 0 mg chol., 195 mg sodium, 30 g carb. (7 g fiber, 5 g sugars), 8 g pro. Exchanges: 1.5 starch, 0.5 carb., 0.5 lean meat, 1 fat.

PER SERVING WITH SUBSTITUTE: Same as above, except 191 cal., 26 g carb. (1 g sugars). Exchanges: 0 carb.

1 | Preheat oven to 300°F. In a bowl whisk together gluten-free all-purpose flour, gluten-free oat flour, flaxseed meal, almond flour, 1 teaspoon cinnamon, and the salt.

2 | In a small bowl stir together the water, vanilla, and, if desired, the stevia sweetener. Add the water mixture to the flour mixture; stir until dough comes together. If necessary, use your clean hands to knead a few times in the bowl to get the dough to combine.

3 | Place a sheet of parchment paper on a baking sheet. Turn out dough onto parchment paper. Top with another sheet of parchment paper. Using a rolling pin and rolling from center to edges, roll dough into a 12-inch square (do not worry if dough cracks slightly). Remove top piece of parchment. In a tiny bowl combine sugar and the ½ teaspoon cinnamon; sprinkle evenly over dough. Using clean hands, press in lightly.

4 | Bake about 30 minutes or until edges are lightly browned. Turn off oven; let cereal sit in oven about 2 hours or until nearly cool (do not cover while it cools). Transfer baking sheet to a wire rack. Cool about 30 minutes more or until completely cooled. Break into small pieces. If desired, serve with milk and berries.

*SUGAR SUBSTITUTE: Choose Splenda Granular. Follow package directions to use amount equivalent to 2 tablespoons sugar.

TO STORE: Store in an airtight container for up to 1 week. If stored cereal softens, preheat oven to 200°F. Spread cereal on a baking sheet. Bake, uncovered, for 10 to 15 minutes or until cereal has regained its crispiness.

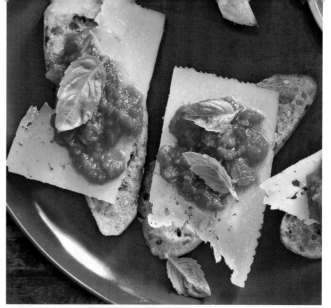

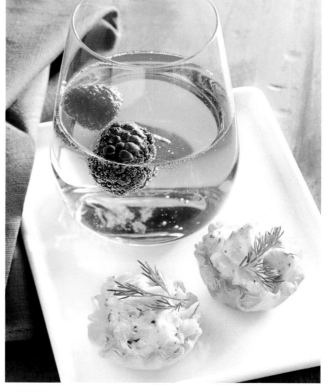

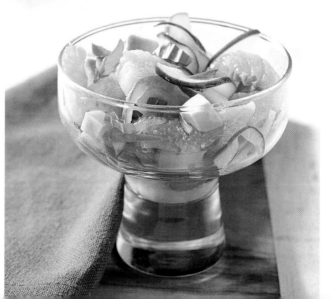

tasty
party bites

'Tis the season to enjoy the company of family and friends.

Whether it's a spread featuring several appetizers or just one or

two, gather everyone around. Serve these lightened versions

of dips, spreads, bruschettas, tarts, and more. And raise a toast

to good health and good cheer.

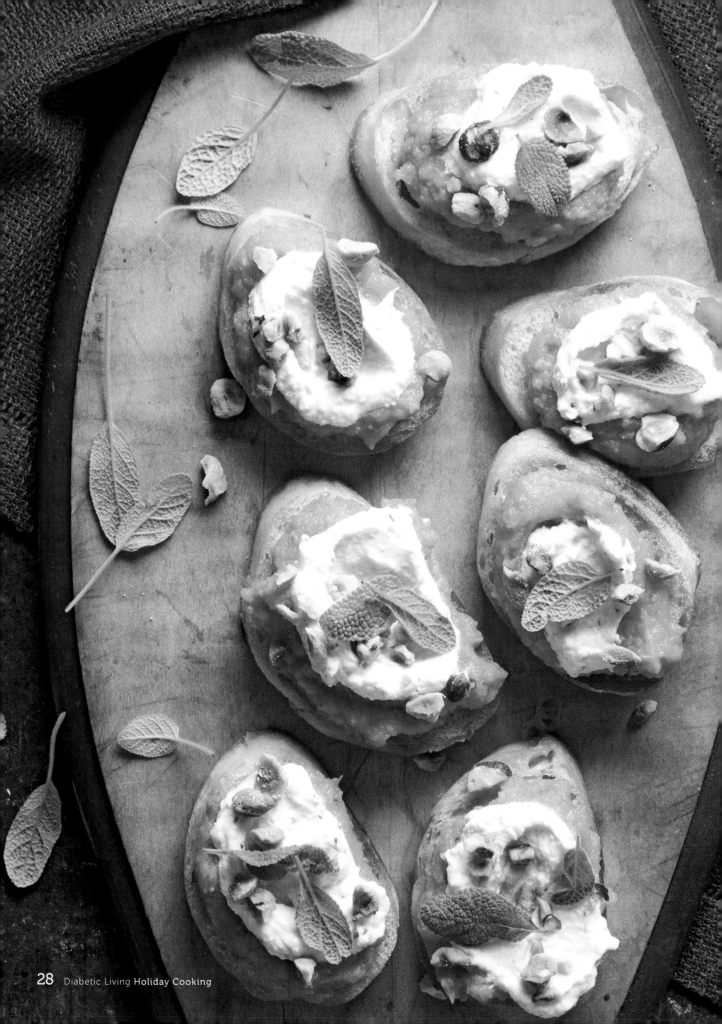

Butternut-Sage Crostini with Ricotta and Hazelnuts

The hint of lemon gives this mellow layered topper a bright flavor. Spread squash and cheese layers to almost cover toasted bread.

SERVINGS 30 (1 crostini each)
CARB. PER SERVING 14 g
PREP 40 minutes **ROAST** 35 minutes **BAKE** 9 minutes

- 1 2-pound butternut squash
- 3/4 cup whole-milk ricotta cheese
- 1 teaspoon finely shredded lemon peel
- 1/2 teaspoon cracked black pepper
- 1/4 teaspoon salt
- Dash cayenne pepper
- 1 tablespoon slivered fresh sage leaves
- 2/3 cup hazelnuts, toasted and chopped
- 2 tablespoons lemon juice
- 1 1-pound loaf baguette-style French bread
- 1/4 cup extra virgin olive oil
- Fresh sage leaves (optional)

1 Preheat oven to 375°F. Line a baking sheet with parchment paper. Cut squash in half lengthwise; scoop out seeds. Place halves, cut sides down, on the prepared baking sheet. Roast squash for 35 to 40 minutes or until tender. Set aside to cool slightly. Increase oven temperature to 400°F.

2 Meanwhile, in a medium bowl stir together ricotta cheese, lemon peel, black pepper, salt, and cayenne pepper; set aside.

3 Scoop flesh from squash halves and transfer to a food processor. Add the 1 tablespoon slivered sage, 1/3 cup of the hazelnuts, and the lemon juice. Cover and process until smooth; set aside.

4 Slice baguette diagonally into 1/2-inch slices. On a very large baking sheet arrange baguette slices in a single layer. Brush slices lightly with half of the olive oil. Bake for 5 to 6 minutes or until slices begin to brown. Turn baguette slices over; brush lightly with the remaining olive oil. Bake for 4 to 5 minutes more or until second sides begin to brown.

5 Thickly spread the butternut squash mixture over baguette slices. Top with ricotta mixture. Sprinkle with the remaining 1/3 cup chopped hazelnuts. Serve warm or at room temperature. If desired, garnish with whole sage leaves.

MAKE-AHEAD DIRECTIONS: Prepare as directed through Step 3. Place ricotta mixture and squash mixture in separate airtight containers; cover. Chill mixtures for up to 24 hours. Let stand at room temperature for 30 minutes before continuing as directed.

PER SERVING: 106 cal., 4 g total fat (1 g sat. fat), 3 mg chol., 139 mg sodium, 14 g carb. (1 g fiber, 1 g sugars), 4 g pro. Exchanges: 1 starch, 0.5 fat.

4 grams pro.

Roma Tomato Jam and Manchego Cheese Bruschetta

Manchego, one of the most popular Spanish cheeses, is made of sheep's milk. Asiago or Pecorino Romano makes a good substitute.

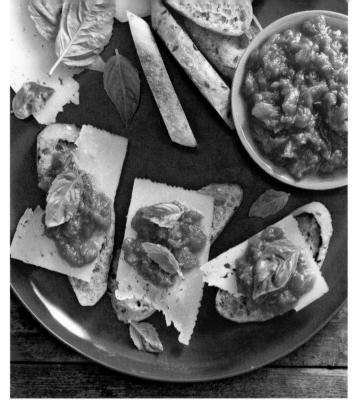

SERVINGS 24 (1 baguette slice, 1 tablespoon jam, and ¼ ounce cheese each)
CARB. PER SERVING 11 g
PREP 45 minutes **ROAST** 1 hour
COOK 1 hour **COOL** 2 hours
BROIL 3 minutes

- 5 pounds roma tomatoes, halved lengthwise
- 2 tablespoons olive oil
- 3 inches stick cinnamon
- 3 whole cardamom pods
- 5 whole cloves
- ½ cup dry red wine (such as Rioja) or cranberry juice
- 3 tablespoons honey
- 2 tablespoons balsamic vinegar
- 24 ½-inch slices baguette-style French bread
- 6 ounces Manchego cheese, thinly sliced

Basil leaves (optional)

PER SERVING: 87 cal., 3 g total fat (1 g sat. fat), 6 mg chol., 200 mg sodium, 11 g carb. (0 g fiber, 2 g sugars), 4 g pro. Exchanges: 0.5 starch, 0.5 medium-fat meat.

1 | Preheat oven to 350°F. Line two 15×10×1-inch baking pans with parchment paper. Place tomatoes, cut sides down, in the prepared baking pans. Brush with oil. Roast about 1 hour or until skins begin to wrinkle and brown. Cool slightly.

2 | Remove skins from tomatoes; carefully scrape out seeds (it's OK if some seeds remain). Place tomatoes, half at a time, in a food processor. Cover and process with on/off pulses until slightly chunky.

3 | For a spice bag, place stick cinnamon, cardamom, and cloves in the center of a double-thick, 6-inch square of 100-percent-cotton cheesecloth. Bring up corners; tie closed with clean kitchen string.

4 | In a large heavy saucepan combine tomatoes, spice bag, wine, honey, and vinegar. Bring to boiling; reduce heat. Simmer, uncovered, about 1 hour or until mixture reaches a thick jamlike consistency, stirring frequently. Remove from heat; remove and discard spice bag. Cool for 2 hours.

5 | Preheat broiler. Place baguette slices on a baking sheet. Broil 3 to 4 inches from the heat about 1 minute or until lightly browned. Top with cheese. Broil about 2 minutes more or until cheese is softened. Top each baguette slice with about 1 tablespoon tomato jam and, if desired, garnish with small basil leaves.

TO STORE: Transfer leftover jam to an airtight container; cover. Chill for up to 1 week or freeze for up to 3 months. If frozen, thaw overnight in the refrigerator.

Polenta Bruschetta

Fried polenta takes the place of traditional toasted French bread. You will need a fork to eat these because polenta is not as sturdy as bread.

SERVINGS 6 (2 slices polenta and 2 tablespoons topping each)
CARB. PER SERVING 12 g
PREP 20 minutes **COOK** 12 minutes

1 16-ounce tube refrigerated cooked polenta

1 tablespoon olive oil

2 roma tomatoes, seeded and chopped

3 tablespoons sliced pitted ripe olives, drained

2 tablespoons snipped fresh basil

1 tablespoon balsamic vinegar

Fresh basil leaves (optional)

PER SERVING: 81 cal., 3 g total fat (0 g sat. fat), 0 mg chol., 216 mg sodium, 12 g carb. (1 g fiber, 1 g sugars), 2 g pro. Exchanges: 1 starch.

1 Trim off and discard the rounded ends of polenta. Bias-slice the remaining polenta into 12 slices, each about $\frac{1}{2}$ inch thick. In a large nonstick skillet heat oil over medium-high heat. Cook polenta slices in batches for 12 to 16 minutes or until golden brown, turning once. Drain on paper towels.

2 Meanwhile, in a small bowl combine tomatoes, olives, the snipped basil, and vinegar. To serve, spoon tomato mixture over polenta slices. If desired, garnish with basil leaves.

MAKE-AHEAD DIRECTIONS: You can cook the polenta slices ahead of time and chill them for up to 24 hours. To reheat the slices, preheat oven to 350°F. Arrange slices in a single layer on a baking sheet. Bake for 5 to 10 minutes or until crisp.

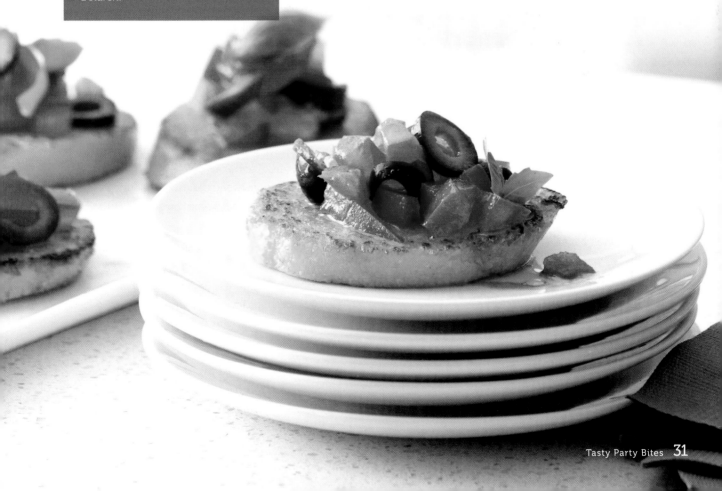

Sweet-Salty Caramelized Onion Spread

Caramelized sweet onions and dried apricots provide the sweetness; crisp-cooked bacon adds saltiness in this cheesy spread.

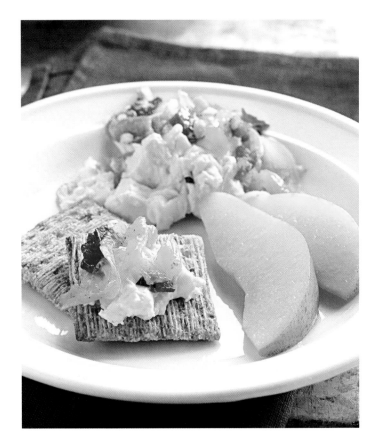

SERVINGS 24 (2 tablespoons spread and 4 apple or pear slices or 4 crackers each)
CARB. PER SERVING 17 g
PREP 25 minutes **BAKE** 15 minutes

¾ cup chopped dried apricots

½ cup dry white wine or light apple juice

3 tablespoons white balsamic vinegar

1 tablespoon honey

4 slices lower-sodium, less-fat bacon, chopped

1 medium sweet onion, cut into thin slivers

2 8-ounce packages reduced-fat cream cheese (Neufchâtel), softened

2 tablespoons fat-free milk

¼ cup snipped fresh Italian (flat-leaf) parsley

Apple slices, pear slices, or whole grain crackers

PER SERVING: 125 cal., 5 g total fat (3 g sat. fat), 15 mg chol., 78 mg sodium, 17 g carb. (2 g fiber, 13 g sugars), 2 g pro. Exchanges: 1 fruit, 1 fat.

1 Preheat oven to 350°F. In a small saucepan combine apricots, wine, and vinegar. Bring to boiling; reduce heat. Simmer gently, covered, for 3 minutes. Remove from heat; stir in honey. Let stand, covered, for 10 minutes, stirring occasionally.

2 Meanwhile, in a medium skillet cook bacon until crisp, stirring occasionally. Using a slotted spoon, transfer bacon to a double thickness of paper towels to drain; reserve drippings in skillet. In the same skillet cook onion in bacon drippings over medium heat for 10 to 12 minutes or until evenly browned and very tender, stirring occasionally. Turn heat down if onion browns too quickly. Remove from the heat and set aside.

3 In a large bowl stir together cream cheese and milk until well combined. Spread cream cheese mixture in the bottom of a 9-inch pie plate or quiche dish.

4 Bake, uncovered, for 10 minutes. Stir cream cheese and spread to an even layer. Top evenly with cooked onions. Bake about 5 minutes more or until cheese is warmed through. Sprinkle with bacon. Drain the apricots; spoon drained apricots evenly over bacon. Sprinkle with parsley. Serve with apple slices, pear slices, or crackers.

Parmesan Dip

For a little color and freshness, sprinkle on snipped fresh chives, dill weed, or thyme just before serving.

SERVINGS 8 (1$\frac{1}{2}$ tablespoons dip and $\frac{3}{4}$ ounce chips each)
CARB. PER SERVING 17 g
START TO FINISH 10 minutes

$\frac{1}{2}$ cup fat-free sour cream

6 tablespoons finely shredded Parmesan cheese

$\frac{1}{4}$ cup fat-free plain Greek yogurt

2 tablespoons snipped fresh chives

1 tablespoon fat-free milk

1 teaspoon Dijon-style mustard

1 teaspoon snipped fresh dill weed or thyme

$\frac{1}{8}$ teaspoon black pepper

6 ounces root vegetable chips (Terra Chips brand or lotus root chips)

1 In a medium bowl combine sour cream, Parmesan cheese, yogurt, chives, milk, mustard, dill, and pepper. Cover and chill until serving time. Serve with root chips.

PER SERVING: 138 cal., 6 g total fat (1 g sat. fat), 4 mg chol., 187 mg sodium, 17 g carb. (3 g fiber, 1 g sugars), 4 g pro. Exchanges: 1 starch, 1 fat.

QUICK TIP
Seek out root vegetable chips in the health food section of the supermarket. Choose the chips that are lowest in fat.

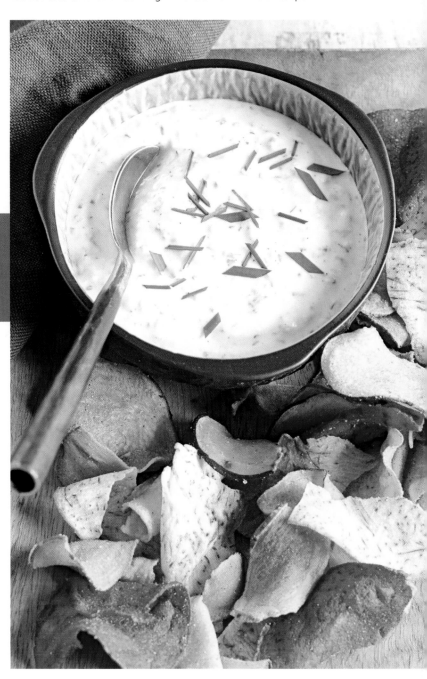

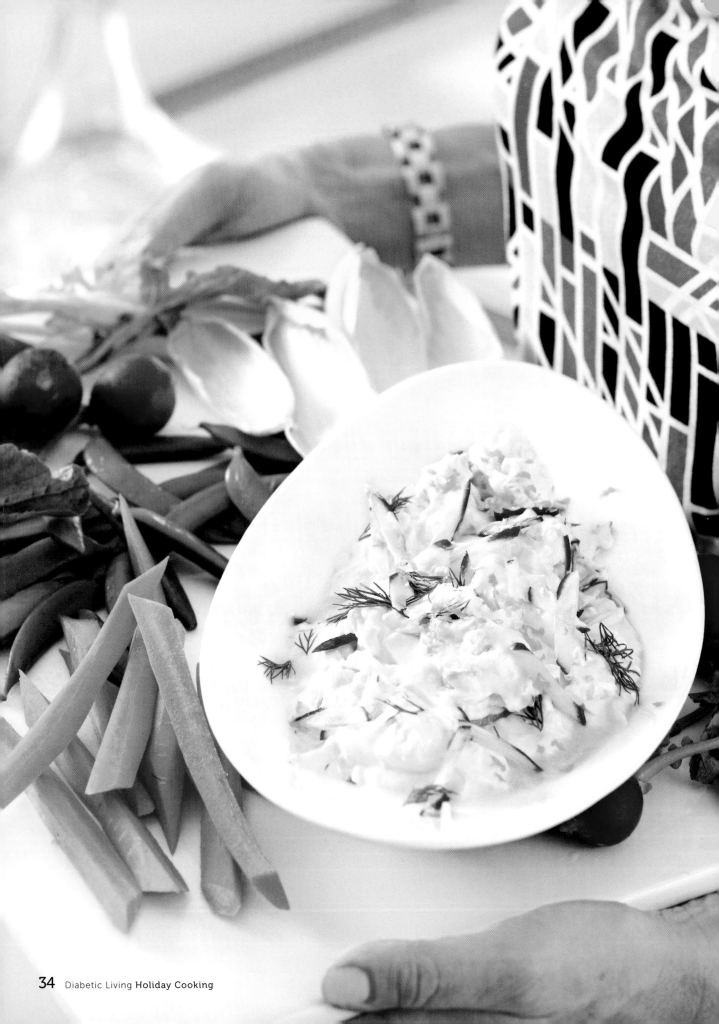

Fresh Radish Dip

Radishes vary in size, so use the scale in the produce section to ensure that you buy 8 ounces for this stir-together dip.

SERVINGS 8 ($^1/4$ cup dip and $^1/2$ cup fresh vegetables each)
CARB. PER SERVING 6 g
START TO FINISH 25 minutes

8 ounces large radishes (about 12), cut into very thin bite-size strips or chopped

$^1/2$ cup light sour cream

$^1/2$ cup crumbled reduced-fat feta cheese (2 ounces)

2 tablespoons snipped fresh dill weed

$^1/2$ teaspoon finely shredded lemon peel

1 tablespoon lemon juice

Fresh dill sprigs (optional)

4 cups radishes, carrot sticks, celery sticks, Belgian endive leaves, and/or fresh snow pea pods

1 In a large bowl stir together radish strips, sour cream, feta cheese, snipped dill, lemon peel, and lemon juice. If desired, garnish with dill sprigs. Serve with fresh vegetables for dipping.

PER SERVING: 56 cal., 3 g total fat (2 g sat. fat), 7 mg chol., 173 mg sodium, 6 g carb. (2 g fiber, 3 g sugars), 3 g pro. Exchanges: 1 vegetable, 0.5 fat.

6 grams carb.

QUICK TIP

This fresh veggie dip is best served immediately after stirring it together. But if you want to get a jump-start on the prep, wash the vegetables that you plan to serve with the dip a few hours before serving and store them in the refrigerator.

Jalapeño, Crab, and Corn Dip

Add more spicy heat to this creamy favorite by stirring in bottled hot pepper sauce.

SERVINGS 24 (2 tablespoons dip and $\frac{1}{2}$ ounce corn chips [6 chips] each)
CARB. PER SERVING 13 g
PREP 30 minutes **COOK** 5 minutes
SLOW COOK 1 hour 30 minutes to 2 hours (low)

- 2 tablespoons butter
- 1 cup frozen whole kernel corn
- $\frac{1}{2}$ cup chopped red sweet pepper (1 small)
- 1 clove garlic, minced
- $\frac{1}{2}$ cup light sour cream
- $\frac{1}{2}$ cup light mayonnaise
- $\frac{1}{2}$ cup sliced pickled jalapeño chile peppers, drained and chopped (see tip, *page 44*)
- 1 teaspoon Worcestershire sauce
- $\frac{1}{2}$ to 1 teaspoon bottled hot pepper sauce (optional)
- 2 6- to 6.5-ounce cans crabmeat, drained, flaked, and cartilage removed
- 1 cup shredded Monterey Jack cheese (4 ounces)
- 2 tablespoons finely shredded Parmesan cheese
- 12 ounces blue or white corn tortilla chips

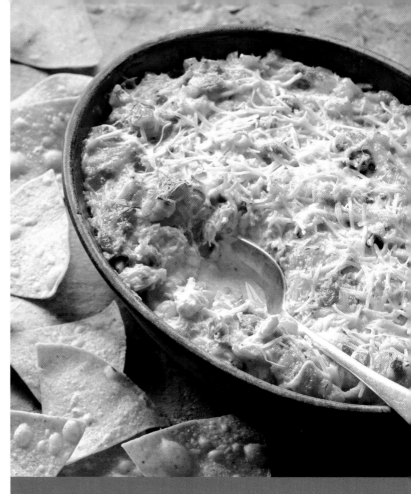

PER SERVING: 132 cal., 7 g total fat (3 g sat. fat), 20 mg chol., 204 mg sodium, 13 g carb. (1 g fiber, 1 g sugars), 4 g pro. Exchanges: 1 starch, 1 fat.

1 In a medium skillet heat butter over medium heat until melted. Add frozen corn, sweet pepper, and garlic; cook and stir for 5 to 8 minutes or until tender.

2 In a medium bowl combine light sour cream, light mayonnaise, jalapeño peppers, Worcestershire sauce, and, if desired, hot pepper sauce. Stir in corn mixture, crabmeat, and Monterey Jack cheese. Transfer crab mixture to a $1\frac{1}{2}$-quart slow cooker.

3 Cover and cook on low-heat setting for $1\frac{1}{2}$ to 2 hours or until heated through. Sprinkle with Parmesan cheese. Serve dip with corn chips.

OVEN DIRECTIONS: Preheat oven to 425°F. Prepare dip through Step 2, except transfer to a $1\frac{1}{2}$-quart baking dish instead of the slow cooker. Sprinkle with Parmesan cheese. Bake, uncovered, about 15 minutes or until golden and bubbly around the edge. Serve with chips.

Herb- and Goat Cheese-Stuffed Mushrooms

Pine nuts toast quickly and can burn easily, so check them often and remove from the oven when just golden.

SERVINGS 24 (1 stuffed mushroom each)
CARB. PER SERVING 3 g
PREP 40 minutes **COOL** 10 minutes **CHILL** 24 hours **BAKE** 15 minutes

24 large fresh cremini mushrooms, about 1½ inches in diameter
2 tablespoons olive oil
¾ teaspoon salt
1 tablespoon butter
1 tablespoon finely chopped shallot
3 cloves garlic, minced
1 teaspoon snipped fresh thyme
¼ cup dry sherry or reduced-sodium chicken broth
¾ cup panko bread crumbs
2 tablespoons snipped fresh chives
2 teaspoons finely shredded lemon peel
1 cup crumbled goat cheese (chèvre) (4 ounces)
¼ cup pine nuts, toasted*
Snipped fresh chives (optional)

1 Remove stems from mushrooms; chop stems and set aside. In a small bowl combine 1 tablespoon of the oil and ¼ teaspoon of the salt; brush mixture onto mushroom caps.

2 For filling, in a large skillet heat the remaining 1 tablespoon oil and the butter over medium-high heat. Add mushroom stems, shallot, garlic, thyme, and the remaining ½ teaspoon salt. Cook and stir for 8 to 10 minutes or until stems are tender and liquid is evaporated. Remove from heat; carefully add sherry. Return to heat; cook until sherry is evaporated, stirring to scrape up any crusty browned bits. Cool for 10 minutes. Stir in panko, 2 tablespoons chives, and lemon peel. Stir in cheese and pine nuts.

3 Place mushroom caps and filling in separate airtight containers. Cover and chill for up to 24 hours.

4 Preheat oven to 400°F. Line a 15×10×1-inch baking pan with parchment paper. Arrange mushroom caps, stemmed sides up, in the prepared baking pan. Generously fill mushroom caps with filling.

5 Bake, uncovered, about 15 minutes or until mushrooms are tender and filling is bubbly around the edges. If desired, sprinkle with additional chives. Serve warm.

***TEST KITCHEN TIP:** To toast nuts, preheat oven to 350°F. Spread nuts in a single layer in a shallow baking pan. Bake for 5 to 10 minutes or until lightly browned, shaking pan once or twice.

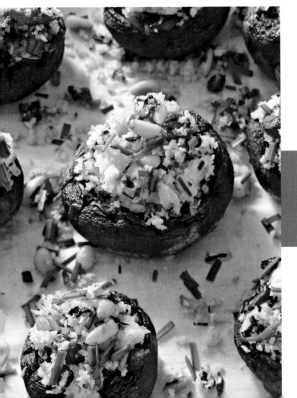

PER SERVING: 57 cal., 4 g total fat (2 g sat. fat), 5 mg chol., 108 mg sodium, 3 g carb. (0 g fiber, 1 g sugars), 2 g pro. Exchanges: 0.5 medium-fat meat, 0.5 fat.

White Wine Cooler

With just three ingredients, this beverage is easy to make and fun to serve.

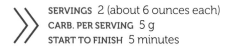

SERVINGS 2 (about 6 ounces each)
CARB. PER SERVING 5 g
START TO FINISH 5 minutes

5 ounces dry white wine, such as Chardonnay, chilled

6 ounces diet cherry-flavor lemon-lime carbonated beverage, chilled

6 fresh raspberries and/or blackberries, frozen

1 | Divide wine between two 6- to 8-ounce wine glasses. Top off each glass with half of the carbonated beverage. Drop raspberries and/or blackberries into glasses. Serve immediately.

PER SERVING: 129 cal., 0 g total fat, 0 mg chol., 30 mg sodium, 5 g carb. (1 g fiber, 2 g sugars), 0 g pro. Exchanges: 2 fat.

Crab Tartlets

Chilling the filling helps the flavors meld before spooning into the shells.

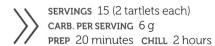

SERVINGS 15 (2 tartlets each)
CARB. PER SERVING 6 g
PREP 20 minutes **CHILL** 2 hours

1 cup cooked crabmeat or one 6-ounce can crabmeat, drained, flaked, and cartilage removed

½ cup light mayonnaise

½ cup light sour cream

2 tablespoons finely chopped red onion or green onion

1 tablespoon snipped fresh dill weed or 1 teaspoon dried dill weed

1 teaspoon finely shredded lemon peel or lime peel

1 teaspoon lemon juice or lime juice

Several dashes bottled hot pepper sauce

⅛ teaspoon salt

⅛ teaspoon black pepper

Dash cayenne pepper (optional)

2 2.1-ounce packages miniature phyllo dough shells (30)

Finely shredded lemon peel (optional)

Fresh dill sprigs (optional)

1 | In a small bowl stir together crab, mayonnaise, sour cream, onion, dill, 1 teaspoon lemon peel, the lemon juice, hot pepper sauce, salt, black pepper, and, if desired, cayenne pepper. Cover and chill for 2 to 24 hours.

2 | Spoon crab mixture into phyllo dough shells. If desired, garnish with lemon peel and dill sprigs.

PER SERVING: 89 cal., 5 g total fat (1 g sat. fat), 13 mg chol., 128 mg sodium, 6 g carb. (0 g fiber, 0 g sugars), 3 g pro. Exchanges: 0.5 starch, 1 fat.

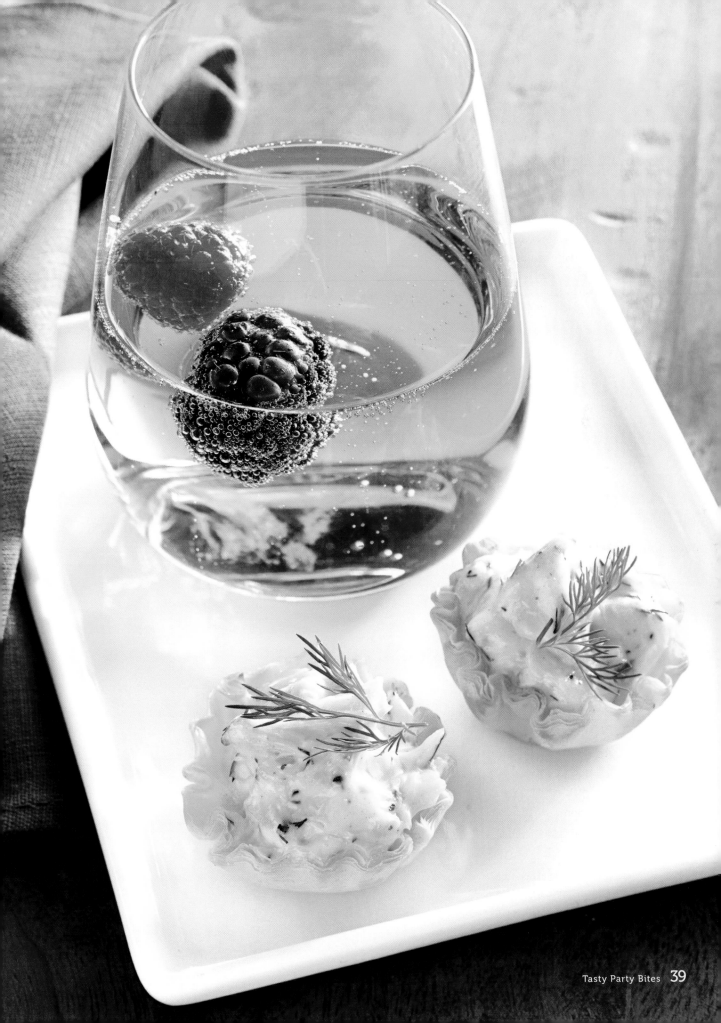

Cauliflower Cheese Bites

These cheesy appetizers are a great way to sneak in more vegetables. Your guests will be surprised that the main ingredient is cauliflower.

SERVINGS 12 (2 bites each)
CARB. PER SERVING 3 g
PREP 30 minutes **BAKE** 15 minutes **BROIL** 2 minutes **COOL** 5 minutes

Nonstick cooking spray

4 cups coarsely chopped fresh cauliflower (about 1 pound)

¼ cup water

½ cup refrigerated or frozen egg product, thawed, or 2 eggs, lightly beaten

2 teaspoons finely snipped fresh rosemary or ½ teaspoon dried rosemary, crushed

3 cloves garlic, minced

¼ teaspoon salt

¼ teaspoon black pepper

6 ounces Fontina cheese, shredded (about 1½ cups)

Fresh rosemary sprigs (optional)

½ cup lower-sodium marinara sauce, warmed (optional)

1 Preheat oven to 375°F. Coat twenty-four 1¾-inch muffin cups with cooking spray; set aside. Place cauliflower in a food processor. Cover and pulse until cauliflower is finely chopped but not pureed (will look similar to broken rice). Transfer cauliflower to a large microwave-safe bowl. Add the water. Cover with vented plastic wrap. Microwave on 100 percent power (high) for 3 to 5 minutes or until cauliflower is almost tender, stirring twice. Let cauliflower cool for 10 minutes, stirring occasionally. Line a strainer or colander with a double layer of 100-percent-cotton cheesecloth. Transfer cauliflower to the lined strainer. Press all the liquid from the cauliflower; discard liquid.

2 In a small bowl combine egg, rosemary, garlic, salt, and pepper. In a medium bowl combine cauliflower and 1¼ cups of the cheese; toss to combine. Add egg mixture to cauliflower mixture; stir until well combined. Divide cauliflower mixture evenly among prepared muffin cups. Press mixture gently into cups with the back of a spoon. Top with remaining cheese.

3 Bake for 15 to 17 minutes or until set. Turn oven to broil. Broil cauliflower bites for 2 to 3 minutes or until tops are golden brown. Cool cauliflower bites in pans on a wire rack for 5 minutes. Run a thin sharp knife around edges of cauliflower bites. Transfer bites to a serving platter. If desired, garnish with rosemary sprigs and serve with warmed marinara sauce.

PER SERVING: 72 cal., 5 g total fat (3 g sat. fat), 16 mg chol., 192 mg sodium, 3 g carb. (1 g fiber, 1 g sugars), 5 g pro. Exchanges: 0.5 vegetable, 0.5 high-fat meat.

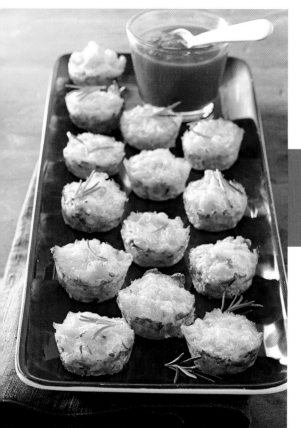

Marinated Veggie and Cheese Roll-Ups

Read labels when selecting tortillas. Choose those that are lowest in carbohydrate and highest in fiber.

SERVINGS 8 (4 slices each)
CARB. PER SERVING 12 g
PREP 25 minutes **MARINATE** 4 hours

- 12 asparagus spears, trimmed
- 2 tablespoons water
- 3 tablespoons white balsamic vinegar
- 2 tablespoons olive oil
- 2 cloves garlic, minced
- 1/8 teaspoon black pepper
- 1/2 of a medium zucchini, cut into 8 long strips
- 1/2 cup bottled roasted red sweet pepper, drained and cut into strips
- 4 green onions, halved lengthwise
- 1 1/2 cups packaged fresh baby spinach leaves
- 4 8-inch low-carb, high-fiber tortillas (such as La Tortilla Factory brand)
- 2 ounces semisoft goat cheese, crumbled, or 1/2 cup reduced-fat crumbled feta cheese

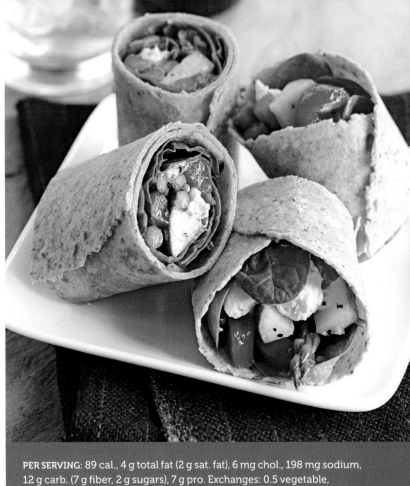

PER SERVING: 89 cal., 4 g total fat (2 g sat. fat), 6 mg chol., 198 mg sodium, 12 g carb. (7 g fiber, 2 g sugars), 7 g pro. Exchanges: 0.5 vegetable, 0.5 starch, 0.5 lean meat, 0.5 fat.

1 Place asparagus in a microwave-safe baking dish with the 2 tablespoons water. Microwave, covered, on 100 percent power (high) for 2 to 4 minutes or until crisp-tender. Drain and cool asparagus.

2 In a small bowl whisk together vinegar, oil, garlic, and black pepper until well combined; set aside. Add asparagus, zucchini, roasted red pepper, and green onions to a large resealable plastic bag. Pour vinegar mixture over vegetables in bag; seal bag. Marinate in the refrigerator for 4 to 6 hours, turning bag occasionally.

3 Drain vegetables, discarding excess marinade. Arrange spinach leaves on top of tortillas. Arrange drained vegetables over spinach, leaving a 1/2-inch border around the edge of each tortilla. Sprinkle vegetables evenly with cheese.

4 Roll up tortillas tightly. Cut each roll-up crosswise into eight slices.

Bacon-Filled Medjool Dates

Each date is a bite of bliss—the saltiness of the crispy bacon and the melty cheese marry with the sweet dates.

SERVINGS 24 (1 date each)
CARB. PER SERVING 21 g
PREP 25 minutes BAKE 12 minutes

6 slices lower-sodium, less-fat bacon

½ cup whole almonds or pecan halves, toasted and chopped

½ cup finely shredded Manchego or Parmesan cheese (2 ounces)

24 unpitted whole Medjool dates (about 1 pound)

3 tablespoons honey

1 teaspoon snipped fresh thyme

PER SERVING: 106 cal., 2 g total fat (1 g sat. fat), 2 mg chol., 46 mg sodium, 21 g carb. (2 g fiber, 18 g sugars), 2 g pro. Exchanges: 1.5 carb., 0.5 fat.

QUICK TIP
Medjool dates are the world's biggest and sweetest dates. This nutrition powerhouse is loaded with antioxidants, fiber, and potassium.

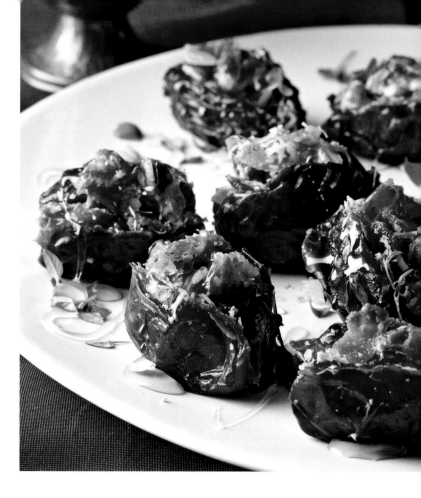

1 | Preheat oven to 375°F. In a large skillet cook bacon over medium heat until crisp. Transfer bacon to paper towels to drain; crumble bacon. In a small bowl stir together the bacon, almonds, and cheese.

2 | Make a slit down one side of each date; spread each date open and remove pit. Spoon about 1 tablespoon of the bacon mixture into each date; press dates to shape around filling (filling will still be exposed).

3 | Arrange dates, filling sides up, on an ungreased baking sheet. Bake for 12 to 15 minutes or until heated through and cheese is lightly browned; cool slightly. Before serving, drizzle warm dates with honey and sprinkle with thyme.

MAKE-AHEAD DIRECTIONS: Prepare dates as directed through Step 2. Place dates in an airtight container; cover. Chill filled dates for up to 2 days. Continue as directed, baking for 15 to 18 minutes.

Mushroom-Chestnut Meatballs with Roasted Pepper Aïoli

If you can't find canned chestnuts, omit them and bump the total to 1$\frac{1}{2}$ cups chopped fresh mushrooms instead.

SERVINGS 12 (2 meatballs and 2 teaspoons aïoli each)
CARB. PER SERVING 6 g
PREP 20 minutes **BAKE** 15 minutes

Nonstick cooking spray

$\frac{3}{4}$ cup chopped fresh button or cremini mushrooms

$\frac{1}{2}$ cup finely chopped onion (1 medium)

$\frac{1}{2}$ cup finely chopped celery (1 stalk)

1 tablespoon olive oil

$\frac{1}{3}$ cup fine dry whole wheat or white bread crumbs

$\frac{1}{4}$ cup refrigerated or frozen egg product, thawed, or 1 egg, lightly beaten

2 teaspoons snipped fresh sage or $\frac{1}{2}$ teaspoon dried sage, crushed

$\frac{1}{4}$ teaspoon black pepper

$\frac{1}{2}$ of a 10-ounce can whole, peeled chestnuts packed in water, rinsed, drained, and finely chopped ($\frac{3}{4}$ cup)*

8 ounces ground pork

8 ounces ground turkey breast

Small fresh sage leaves (optional)

1 recipe Roasted Pepper Aïoli

1 Preheat oven to 350°F. Line a 15×10×1-inch baking pan with foil. Coat foil with cooking spray; set aside. In a large skillet cook mushrooms, onion, and celery in hot oil over medium heat about 5 minutes or until tender, stirring occasionally.

2 In a large bowl combine bread crumbs, egg, sage, and black pepper. Stir in mushroom mixture and chestnuts. Add pork and turkey; mix well.

3 Shape meat mixture into 24 meatballs about 1$\frac{1}{4}$ inch in diameter. Place meatballs in the prepared pan. Bake for 15 to 20 minutes or until done in centers (165°F). Drain on paper towels; transfer to a serving platter and keep warm. Serve warm meatballs with Roasted Pepper Aïoli for dipping. If desired, garnish platter with fresh sage leaves.

ROASTED PEPPER AÏOLI: In a blender or food processor combine $\frac{1}{4}$ cup plain fat-free Greek yogurt; 3 tablespoons chopped bottled roasted red sweet pepper, drained; $\frac{1}{2}$ teaspoon finely shredded lemon peel; 1 tablespoon lemon juice; 1 clove garlic, minced; and $\frac{1}{8}$ teaspoon freshly ground black pepper. Cover and blend or process until smooth.

*TEST KITCHEN TIP: If you can't find canned chestnuts, omit them and increase the fresh mushrooms to 1$\frac{1}{2}$ cups.

PER SERVING: 109 cal., 5 g total fat (1 g sat. fat), 22 mg chol., 72 mg sodium, 6 g carb. (1 g fiber, 1 g sugars), 10 g pro. Exchanges: 0.5 starch, 1 lean meat, 0.5 fat.

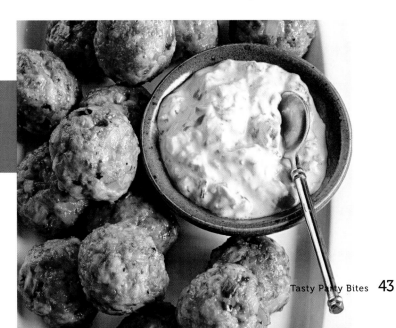

Scallop-Grapefruit Ceviche with Vegetables

Ceviche, a popular Latin America medley, is traditionally made of raw fish cured in citrus juice. Here the scallops are cooked.

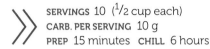

SERVINGS 10 (½ cup each)
CARB. PER SERVING 10 g
PREP 15 minutes **CHILL** 6 hours

- 12 ounces fresh or frozen sea scallops
- 3 tablespoons olive oil
- ⅓ cup grapefruit juice
- 3 tablespoons white balsamic vinegar
- 2 cloves garlic, minced
- ¼ teaspoon salt
- ⅛ teaspoon black pepper
- 1 medium red sweet pepper, cut into thin bite-size strips
- 1 small zucchini, trimmed, halved lengthwise, and thinly sliced
- ½ of a medium red onion, cut into thin slivers
- 1 small fresh jalapeño or serrano chile pepper, seeded and chopped*
- 1 medium red grapefruit, peeled and sectioned
- 1 medium avocado, halved, seeded, peeled, and chopped
- 3 tablespoons thinly sliced fresh basil

1 Thaw scallops, if frozen. Rinse scallops with cold water; pat dry with paper towels. In a large skillet cook scallops in 1 tablespoon of the oil over medium-high heat for 2 to 3 minutes or until browned, turning once. Transfer to a cutting board. Let cool about 5 minutes. Cut scallops in half horizontally.

2 In a large bowl whisk together remaining 2 tablespoons oil, the grapefruit juice, vinegar, garlic, salt, and black pepper. Add scallops, sweet pepper, zucchini, red onion, and jalapeño pepper. Toss gently to coat. Cover and chill for 6 to 8 hours, stirring occasionally.

3 Just before serving, add grapefruit sections and avocado to the scallop mixture. Stir gently to combine.

4 Using a slotted spoon, divide mixture evenly among six martini glasses. Sprinkle with basil just before serving.

***TEST KITCHEN TIP:** Because chile peppers contain volatile oils that can burn your skin and eyes, avoid direct contact with them as much as possible. When working with chile peppers, wear plastic or rubber gloves. If your bare hands do touch the peppers, wash your hands and nails well with soap and warm water.

10 grams carb.

PER SERVING: 113 cal., 6 g total fat (1 g sat. fat), 8 mg chol., 195 mg sodium, 10 g carb. (2 g fiber, 5 g sugars), 5 g pro. Exchanges: 0.5 vegetable, 0.5 carb., 0.5 lean meat, 1 fat.

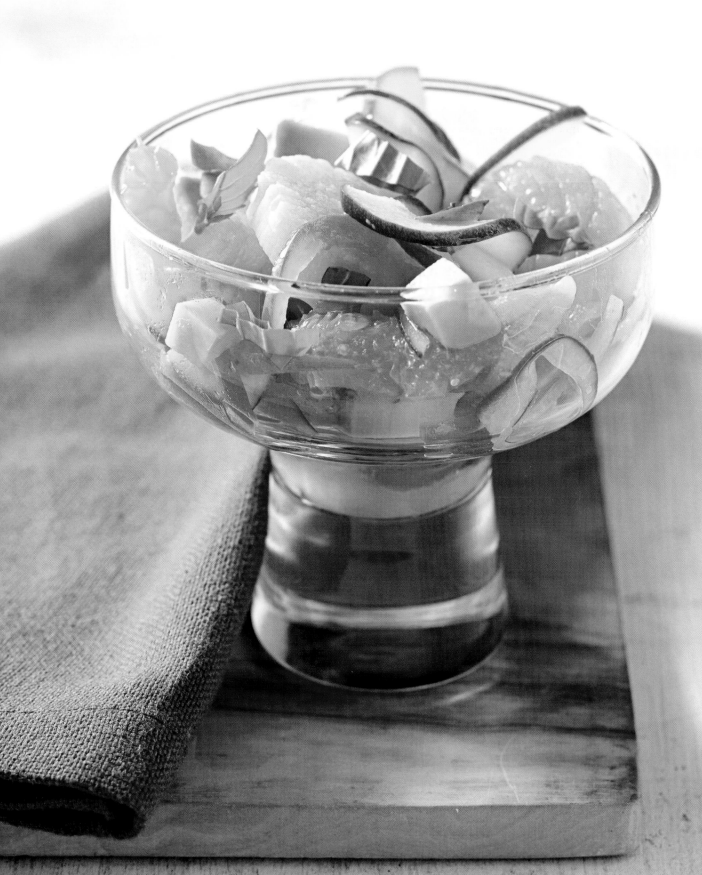

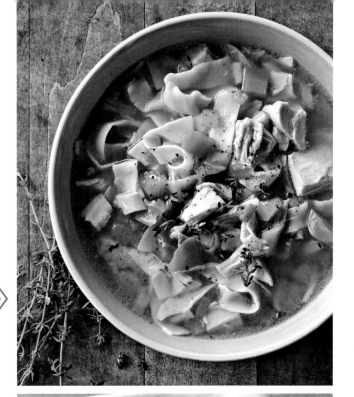

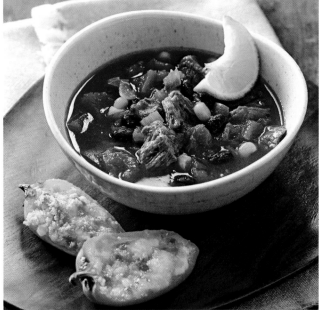

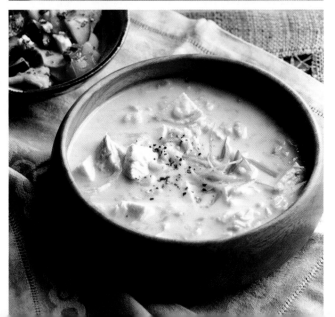

comforting
soups and stews

Something sensational happens when the aroma of a simmering

pot of soup wafts through the house—the promise that a warm

and wonderful bowl of homemade goodness is on the way. Mix

up your repertoire of favorite bowls with these new recipes—

each lightened up and full of flavor.

Turkey Meatball and Tomatillo White Chili

For the leanest option, use ground turkey breast.

SERVINGS 6 (1¹/₃ cups chili and
1 tablespoon sour cream each)
CARB. PER SERVING 33 g
PREP 25 minutes BAKE 20 minutes
COOK 21 minutes

- 2 egg whites
- 1/3 cup fine dry whole wheat or regular bread crumbs
- 1/4 cup snipped fresh cilantro
- 4 cloves garlic, minced
- 1/2 teaspoon paprika
- 1 pound lean ground turkey
- 1 small red onion, cut into thin wedges
- 1 tablespoon canola oil
- 1 teaspoon cumin seeds, crushed
- 8 fresh tomatillos (about 1 pound)
- 1 15-ounce can no-salt-added cannellini beans (white kidney beans), rinsed and drained
- 1 14.75-ounce can cream-style corn
- 1 cup reduced-sodium chicken broth
- 1 cup water
- 1 to 2 fresh serrano chile peppers, seeded, if desired, and finely chopped (see tip, *page 59*)
- 1/2 cup light sour cream (optional)
- 1 fresh serrano chile pepper, seeded and very thinly sliced (optional)
- 1/3 cup coarsely snipped fresh cilantro

PER SERVING: 306 cal., 11 g total fat
(2 g sat. fat), 56 mg chol.,
446 mg sodium, 33 g carb. (6 g fiber,
7 g sugars), 22 g pro. Exchanges:
1 vegetable, 1.5 starch, 2.5 lean meat,
1 fat.

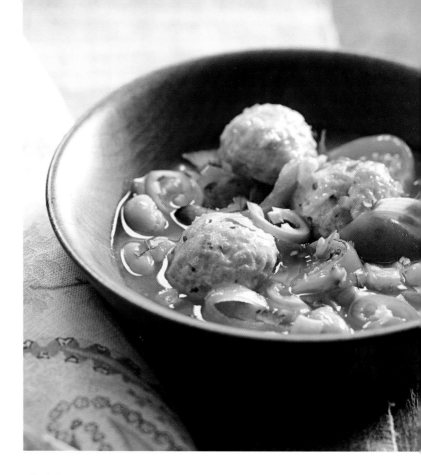

1 Preheat oven to 350°F. In a large bowl beat egg whites with a fork. Stir in bread crumbs, 1/4 cup cilantro, garlic, and paprika. Add turkey; mix well. Shape mixture into about eighteen 1¹/₂-inch meatballs. Place meatballs in a foil-lined 15×10×1-inch baking pan. Bake about 20 minutes or until no longer pink (165°F). Set aside.

2 In a 4-quart Dutch oven cook onion in hot oil over medium heat for 6 to 8 minutes or until tender and just starting to brown, stirring occasionally. Add cumin seeds; cook and stir for 30 seconds more. Transfer onion mixture to a bowl; set aside.

3 Remove husks from fresh tomatillos. Wash tomatillos; trim and cut each tomatillo into six wedges. Add fresh tomatillos to the same Dutch oven. Cook over medium-high heat for 3 to 5 minutes or until tomatillos are softened and starting to brown, stirring occasionally.

4 Return onion mixture to the pan with tomatillos. Add beans, corn, broth, water, and chopped serrano peppers. Bring to boiling; reduce heat. Simmer, uncovered, for 10 minutes to blend flavors. Add cooked meatballs; cook for 1 to 2 minutes or until meatballs are heated through.

5 To serve, ladle hot soup into six soup bowls. If desired, top with sour cream and garnish with sliced serrano pepper. Sprinkle with 1/3 cup cilantro.

Tuscan Chicken, Bean, and Kale Soup with Crispy Haricots Verts

Tuscan kale, also known as lacinato kale or dinosaur kale, is loaded with vitamins A, C, and K. Expect its sturdy leaves to wilt slightly when cooked.

SERVINGS 6 (1$^1/_3$ cups soup and 2 ounces beans each)
CARB. PER SERVING 28 g
PREP 50 minutes   BAKE 9 minutes

- 2 teaspoons light butter with canola oil
- ½ cup chopped onion (1 medium)
- ½ cup coarsely chopped carrot (1 medium)
- ½ cup coarsely chopped celery (1 stalk)
- 2 links cooked sweet Italian-style chicken sausage, thinly sliced
- 2 cloves garlic, minced
- ¼ teaspoon salt
- 4 cups unsalted chicken stock
- 1 15-ounce can no-salt-added cannellini beans (white kidney beans), rinsed and drained
- ½ cup canned no-salt-added diced tomatoes, undrained
- 4 cups torn fresh Tuscan kale
- 1 tablespoon snipped fresh thyme
- 2 teaspoons snipped fresh oregano
- 1 recipe Crispy Haricots Verts

1 | In a 4-quart Dutch oven melt butter over medium heat. Add onion, carrot, and celery; cook for 5 to 7 minutes or until onion is translucent. Add chicken sausage, garlic, and salt; cook about 4 minutes more or until sausage is lightly browned.

2 | Stir in chicken stock, cannellini beans, and tomatoes. Bring to boiling. Add kale, thyme, and oregano. Reduce heat. Simmer, uncovered, for 5 minutes. Ladle into six soup bowls. Serve with Crispy Haricot Verts.

CRISPY HARICOTS VERTS: Preheat oven to 450°F. Line a 15×10×1-inch baking pan with foil; set aside. Trim 12 ounces thin fresh green beans (haricots verts). Rinse beans and pat dry with paper towels; set aside. In a shallow dish use a fork to beat together 1 egg, 1 egg white, and 1 tablespoon Dijon-style mustard. Place $^2/_3$ cup fine dry whole wheat bread crumbs in a second shallow dish. Dip green beans into egg mixture, then into bread crumbs, turning to coat all sides. Place green beans on prepared baking pan. Coat green beans with nonstick cooking spray. Bake for 9 to 11 minutes or until coating is golden brown.

PER SERVING: 232 cal., 5 g total fat (1 g sat. fat), 53 mg chol., 623 mg sodium, 28 g carb. (6 g fiber, 5 g sugars), 17 g pro. Exchanges: 2 vegetable, 1 starch, 1.5 lean meat, 0.5 fat.

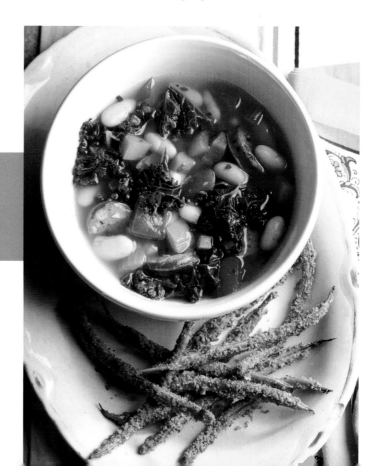

Old-Fashioned Chicken Noodle Soup

Homemade Egg Noodles take this humble bowl to gourmet status. If you are in a hurry, dried egg noodles make a quick and delicious option.

SERVINGS 8 (1$^1/_3$ cups each)
CARB. PER SERVING 29 g
PREP 25 minutes COOK 1 hour 40 minutes

- 1   3$^1/_2$- to 4-pound broiler-fryer chicken, cut up, or 3 pounds meaty chicken pieces (breast halves, thighs, and/or drumsticks)
- $^1/_2$ cup chopped onion (1 medium)
- 1   teaspoon salt
- 1   teaspoon dried thyme, sage, or basil, crushed
- $^1/_4$ teaspoon black pepper
- 2   bay leaves
- 2   cloves garlic, peeled and halved
- 8   cups water
- 1   cup chopped carrots (2 medium)
- 1   cup chopped celery (2 stalks)
- 2   cups Homemade Egg Noodles (see recipe, *page 51*) or 6 ounces dried egg noodles
- 1   tablespoon snipped fresh thyme, sage, or basil (optional)

PER SERVING: 275 cal., 6 g total fat (1 g sat. fat), 136 mg chol., 535 mg sodium, 29 g carb. (2 g fiber, 2 g sugars), 26 g pro. Exchanges: 0.5 vegetable, 1.5 starch, 3 lean meat.

1 | In a 6- to 8-quart Dutch oven combine chicken, onion, salt, dried thyme, pepper, bay leaves, and garlic. Pour the water over all. Bring to boiling; reduce heat. Simmer, covered, about 1$^1/_2$ hours or until chicken is very tender.

2 | Remove chicken from broth. When cool enough to handle, remove meat from bones. Discard bones and skin. Cut meat into bite-size pieces; set aside. Discard bay leaves. Skim fat from broth.

3 | Bring broth to boiling. Stir in carrots and celery. Simmer, covered, for 7 minutes. Add Homemade Egg Noodles, stirring to combine. Simmer, covered, for 3 to 5 minutes more or until noodles are tender. Stir in chicken pieces and, if desired, fresh thyme; heat through. Ladle into eight soup bowls.

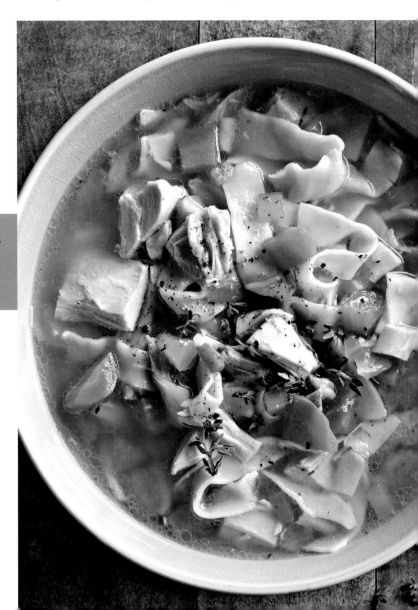

Homemade Egg Noodles

Making homemade noodles is eaiser than you think. A rolling pin and a steady arm are all you need for rolling them out.

SERVINGS 8 ($^3/_4$ cup each)
CARB. PER SERVING 26 g
PREP 50 minutes STAND 20 minutes

- 2 cups flour
- $^1/_2$ teaspoon salt
- 2 egg yolks
- 1 egg
- $^1/_3$ cup water
- 1 teaspoon vegetable oil or olive oil

Flour

1 In a large bowl stir together 1$^3/_4$ cups of the flour and the salt. Make a well in the center of the flour mixture. In a small bowl combine egg yolks, whole egg, the water, and oil. Add egg mixture to flour mixture; stir until mixture forms dough.

2 Sprinkle a clean kneading surface with the remaining $^1/_4$ cup flour. Turn dough out onto the floured surface. Knead until dough is smooth and elastic (10 minutes total kneading time). Cover and let the dough rest for 10 minutes. Divide the dough into four equal portions.

3 On a lightly floured surface roll each dough portion into a 12-inch square (about $^1/_{16}$ inch thick). Lightly dust both sides of the dough square with additional flour. Let stand, uncovered, about 20 minutes. (Or using a pasta machine, pass each dough portion through machine according to manufacturer's directions until dough is $^1/_{16}$ inch thick, dusting dough with flour as needed. Let stand, uncovered, for 20 minutes.) Loosely roll dough square into a spiral; cut crosswise into $^1/_4$-inch-wide strips. Unroll strips to separate; cut strips into 2- to 3-inch-long pieces. Add to simmering soup and cook for 3 minutes or until tender. If using noodles for another purpose, cook noodle pieces in a large amount of boiling lightly salted water for 2 to 3 minutes or until tender; drain well. (Or place noodle pieces in a resealable plastic bag or an airtight container and store in the refrigerator for up to 1 day before cooking.) Makes about 1 pound of fresh pasta.

PER SERVING: 148 cal., 3 g total fat (1 g sat. fat), 69 mg chol., 157 mg sodium, 26 g carb. (1 g fiber, 0 g sugars), 5 g pro. Exchanges: 1.5 starch.

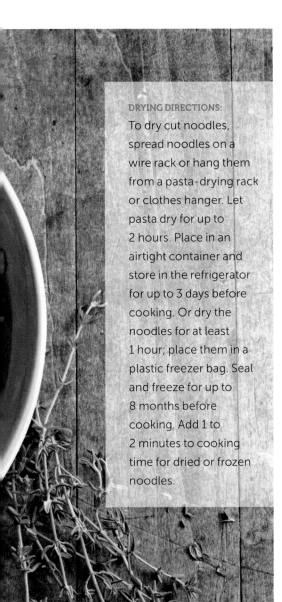

DRYING DIRECTIONS:
To dry cut noodles, spread noodles on a wire rack or hang them from a pasta-drying rack or clothes hanger. Let pasta dry for up to 2 hours. Place in an airtight container and store in the refrigerator for up to 3 days before cooking. Or dry the noodles for at least 1 hour; place them in a plastic freezer bag. Seal and freeze for up to 8 months before cooking. Add 1 to 2 minutes to cooking time for dried or frozen noodles.

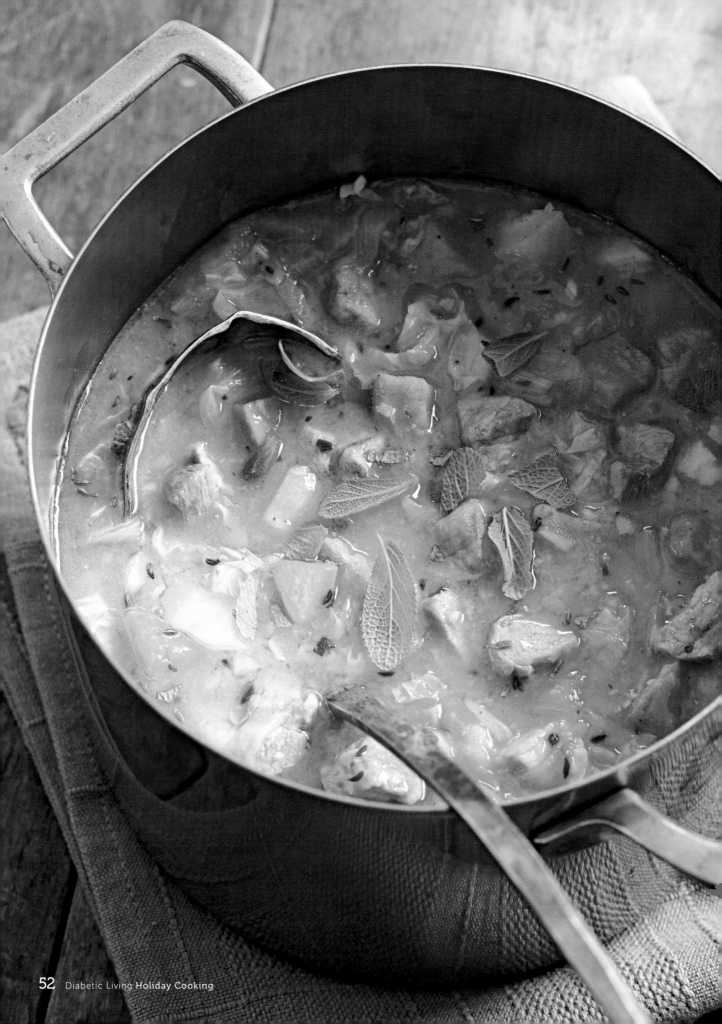

German Pork and Winter Vegetable Stew

Savoy cabbage has sweet, tender green leaves. If it's not available in your supermarket, try napa cabbage or traditional cabbage.

SERVINGS 6 (1$^1/_3$ cups stew and 1 tablespoon topping each)
CARB. PER SERVING 29 g
PREP 25 minutes   COOK 22 minutes

1$^1/_2$ pounds boneless pork sirloin roast

1   large onion, cut into thin wedges (1 cup)

2   tablespoons canola oil

1   tablespoon snipped fresh sage or 1 teaspoon dried sage, crushed

1   teaspoon caraway seeds, crushed

1   32-ounce carton reduced-sodium chicken broth

14   ounces parsnips, peeled, halved lengthwise, and cut crosswise into $^1/_2$-inch-thick slices (2$^1/_2$ cups)

1   bay leaf

12   ounces sweet potatoes, peeled and cut into 1-inch cubes (2 cups)

$^1/_2$ cup cold water

3   tablespoons flour

4   cups shredded savoy cabbage

$^1/_3$ cup light sour cream

2   tablespoons coarse-ground mustard

Fresh sage leaves (optional)

1 | Trim fat from pork. Cut pork into 1-inch cubes. In a 5- to 6-quart Dutch oven cook half the pork and half the onions in 1 tablespoon of the oil over medium-high heat for 4 to 6 minutes or until pork is browned, stirring occasionally. Transfer pork mixture to a medium bowl. Repeat with remaining pork, remaining onion, and remaining oil. Stir in dried sage, if using, and caraway seeds. Cook and stir for 30 seconds more. Return the first batch of pork and onion to the Dutch oven.

2 | Add broth, parsnips, and bay leaf to pork mixture. Bring to boiling; reduce heat. Simmer, covered, for 5 minutes. Add sweet potatoes and simmer, covered, about 10 minutes more or until pork and vegetables are tender.

3 | In a small bowl whisk together water and flour until smooth. Add to pork mixture along with cabbage and, if using, fresh sage. Cook and stir until slightly thickened and bubbly; cook and stir for 1 minute more.

4 | Remove bay leaf and discard. To serve, ladle stew into six soup bowls. For topping, in a small bowl combine sour cream and mustard. Divide evenly among servings. If desired, garnish with fresh sage leaves.

PER SERVING: 328 cal., 10 g total fat (2 g sat. fat), 82 mg chol., 534 mg sodium, 29 g carb. (6 g fiber, 7 g sugars), 30 g pro. Exchanges: 1.5 vegetable, 1.5 starch, 3 lean meat, 1 fat.

10 grams fat

Roasted Beet Soup with Pork Dumplings

If you have an immersion blender, skip the blending or processing step and blend the roasted beet mixture, evaporated milk, broth, and water in the Dutch oven.

SERVINGS 6 (1 cup soup and 3 dumplings each)
CARB. PER SERVING 35 g
PREP 50 minutes ROAST 1 hour

1½ pounds beets, peeled and cut into wedges

1 medium onion, cut into wedges

1 medium Granny Smith apple, peeled, cored, and cut into wedges

4 cloves garlic, peeled

2 teaspoons olive oil

¼ teaspoon salt

⅛ teaspoon ground white pepper

1 cup evaporated fat-free milk

2 cups reduced-sodium chicken broth

1 cup water

2 teaspoons snipped fresh thyme

2 tablespoons fat-free sour cream

Snipped fresh thyme (optional)

1 recipe Pork Dumplings

PER SERVING: 281 cal., 10 g total fat (3 g sat. fat), 25 mg chol., 574 mg sodium, 35 g carb. (4 g fiber, 15 g sugars), 13 g pro. Exchanges: 2 vegetable, 1.5 starch, 1 medium-fat meat, 1 fat.

1 Preheat oven to 375°F. Line a large baking sheet with foil; set aside. In a large bowl combine beets, onion, apple, garlic, olive oil, salt, and white pepper. Spread in an even layer on the prepared baking sheet. Roast about 1 hour or until beets are tender.

2 Transfer roasted beet mixture to a blender or food processor. Add evaporated milk. Cover and blend or process until nearly smooth. In a 4- to 6-quart Dutch oven combine pureed beet mixture, broth, the water, and the 2 teaspoons thyme. Bring to boiling; reduce heat. Simmer, uncovered, for 5 to 10 minutes or until soup is thickened to desired consistency. Ladle into six soup bowls. Top individual servings with sour cream. If desired, sprinkle with additional thyme. Serve with Pork Dumplings.

PORK DUMPLINGS: For filling, in a medium skillet cook 4 ounces ground pork over medium heat until no longer pink, breaking up meat as it cooks; drain off fat. Cool slightly. In a medium bowl combine pork, ½ cup finely chopped cabbage, 2 tablespoons tub cream cheese spread with chive and onion (1 ounce), 2 tablespoons finely chopped onion, 2 teaspoons snipped fresh thyme, and ¼ teaspoon black pepper. For dumplings, use 18 wonton wrappers. Place about 2 teaspoons filling in the center of a wonton wrapper. Lightly brush edges of wrapper with water, fold wrapper in half over filling, and pleat edges together. (Or bring two opposite corners together in center; repeat with the remaining two opposite corners.) (Keep remaining wrappers covered with a slightly damp paper towel to prevent them from drying out.) Repeat with remaining filling and wrappers. Bring a large pot of water to simmering. Add dumplings. Simmer, uncovered, about 1 minute or just until dumplings float. Drain well. In a large nonstick skillet heat 1½ teaspoons olive oil over medium-high heat. Add half of the dumplings and cook about 2 minutes or until browned; turn dumplings and cook for 1 to 2 minutes more or until browned on second sides. Repeat with 1½ teaspoons olive oil and remaining dumplings.

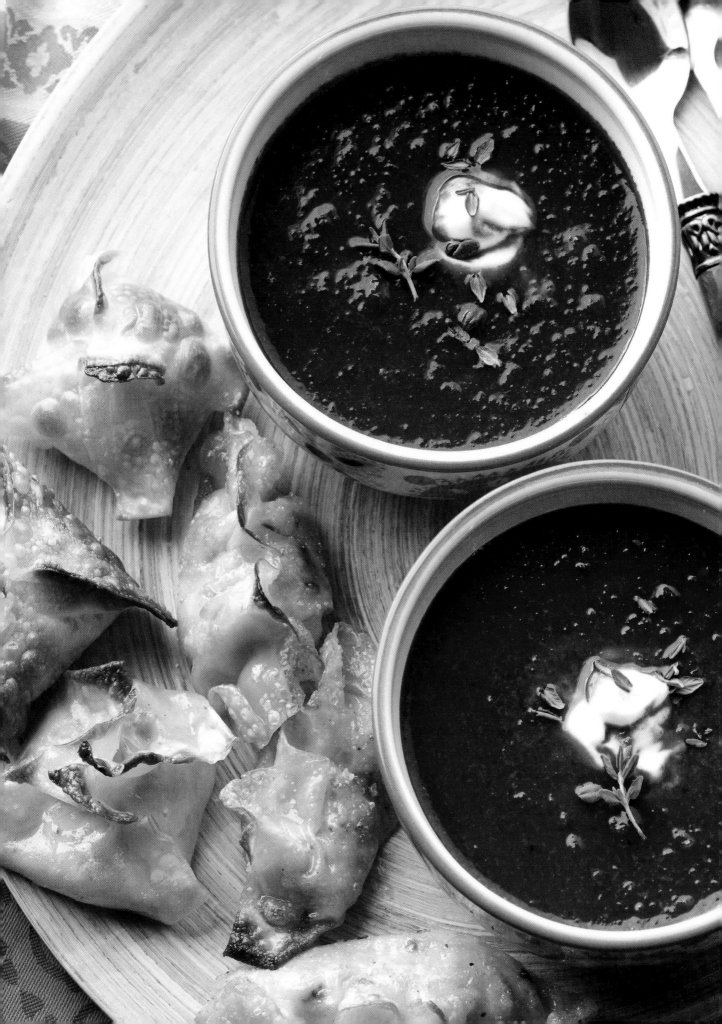

Mexican Shredded Beef Soup with Stuffed Mini Peppers

Pair the extra mini sweet peppers with traditional hummus as a protein-packed snack.

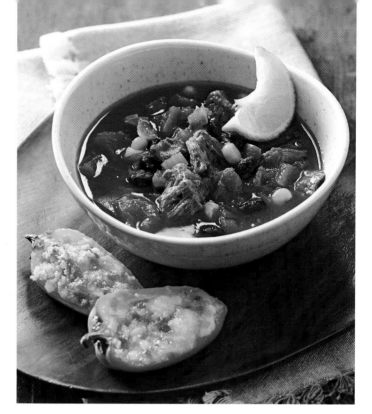

SERVINGS 6 (1 cup soup and 2 pepper halves each)
CARB. PER SERVING 27 g
PREP 40 minutes
COOK 1 hour 35 minutes
BAKE 12 minutes

- 1 pound beef chuck eye steak
- 2 teaspoons olive oil
- 1 cup chopped onion (1 large)
- 1 teaspoon paprika
- ½ teaspoon salt
- ½ teaspoon ground cumin
- ¼ teaspoon black pepper
- 2 14.5-ounce cans no-salt-added diced tomatoes, undrained
- 1 14.5-ounce can 50%-less-sodium beef broth
- 1 15-ounce can no-salt-added black beans, rinsed and drained
- 1 large green or red sweet pepper, seeded and cut into bite-size pieces
- ½ cup frozen whole kernel corn
- 2 teaspoons snipped fresh cilantro
- 1 recipe Stuffed Mini Peppers
  Lime wedges (optional)

PER SERVING: 269 cal., 9 g total fat (4 g sat. fat), 46 mg chol., 515 mg sodium, 27 g carb. (8 g fiber, 9 g sugars), 22 g pro. Exchanges: 2 vegetable, 1 starch, 2 lean meat, 1 fat.

1 If necessary, trim fat from beef; cut beef into 2-inch pieces. In a 4-quart Dutch oven heat oil over medium-high heat. Add beef; cook and stir until browned on all sides. Add onion, paprika, salt, cumin, and black pepper. Cook and stir for 2 minutes more. Add tomatoes and broth, stirring to scrape up the browned bits from bottom of pan. Bring to boiling; reduce heat. Simmer, covered, about 1½ hours or until beef is tender.

2 Transfer beef to a cutting board; let cool slightly. Using two forks, pull meat apart into shreds. Return beef to Dutch oven. Add black beans, sweet pepper, and corn. Bring soup to boiling; reduce heat. Simmer, covered, about 5 minutes more or just until sweet pepper is tender. Stir in cilantro. Ladle into six soup bowls. Serve with Stuffed Mini Peppers. If desired, serve with lime wedges.

STUFFED MINI PEPPERS: Preheat oven to 375°F. Line a baking sheet with foil; set aside. In a small bowl toss together ½ cup crumbled queso fresco (2 ounces), ¼ cup shredded part-skim mozzarella cheese (1 ounce), and 2 tablespoons finely chopped jarred pimiento. Halve and seed 6 miniature red, yellow, and/or green sweet peppers. Stuff pepper halves with cheese mixture, mounding mixture slightly. Sprinkle 1 tablespoon whole wheat panko bread crumbs on top of cheese mixture in each pepper half. Lightly coat top of panko with nonstick cooking spray. Place peppers on prepared baking sheet. Bake for 12 to 15 minutes or until golden brown on top.

Orange- and Saffron-Scented Fish Soup

Saffron is the stigma (threadlike filaments) of the flowering crocus. Because it is labor-intensive to produce, saffron is expensive to buy. But the good news is a little bit of this golden spice with fragrant flavor goes a long way.

SERVINGS 6 (1½ cups each)
CARB. PER SERVING 11 g
PREP 25 minutes SLOW COOK 8 to 10 hours (low) or 4 to 5 hours (high) + 20 minutes (high)

- 3 cups reduced-sodium vegetable broth
- 1 14.5-ounce can no-salt-added diced tomatoes, undrained
- 1 cup finely chopped fennel (1 medium)
- ¾ cup finely chopped red sweet pepper (1 medium)
- ½ cup finely chopped celery (1 stalk)
- ½ cup dry white wine or reduced-sodium vegetable broth
- 1 teaspoon finely shredded orange peel
- ½ cup orange juice
- ¼ cup finely chopped shallots (2 medium)
- 1 fresh serrano or other chile pepper, seeded and finely chopped (see tip, *page 59*)
- 1 bay leaf
- ½ teaspoon salt
- 1 pound fresh or frozen skinless cod, orange roughy, and/or haddock fillets
- 8 ounces fresh or frozen skinless salmon fillets
- ⅛ teaspoon saffron threads, crumbled, or dash ground saffron
- ½ cup snipped fresh parsley

1 In a 3½- or 4-quart slow cooker combine broth, tomatoes, fennel, sweet pepper, celery, wine, orange peel, orange juice, shallots, chile pepper, bay leaf, and salt. Cover and cook on low-heat setting for 8 to 10 hours or on high-heat setting for 4 to 5 hours or until vegetables are tender.

2 Meanwhile, thaw fish, if frozen. Rinse fish; pat dry with paper towels. Cut into 1- to 1½-inch pieces. Cover and chill until needed.

3 If using low-heat setting, turn cooker to high-heat setting. Remove and discard bay leaf. Gently stir in fish and saffron. Cover and cook about 20 minutes more or until fish flakes easily when tested with a fork. Stir in parsley. Ladle into six soup bowls.

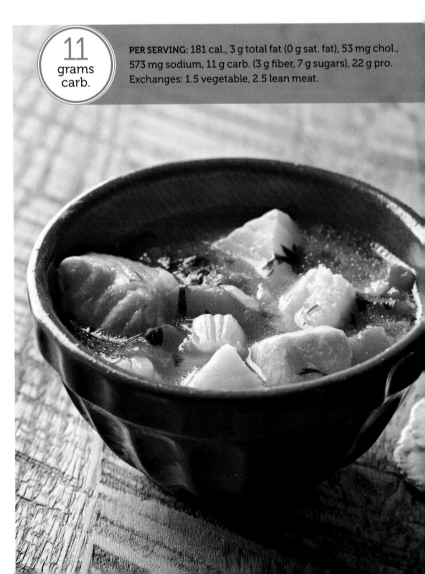

11 grams carb.

PER SERVING: 181 cal., 3 g total fat (0 g sat. fat), 53 mg chol., 573 mg sodium, 11 g carb. (3 g fiber, 7 g sugars), 22 g pro. Exchanges: 1.5 vegetable, 2.5 lean meat.

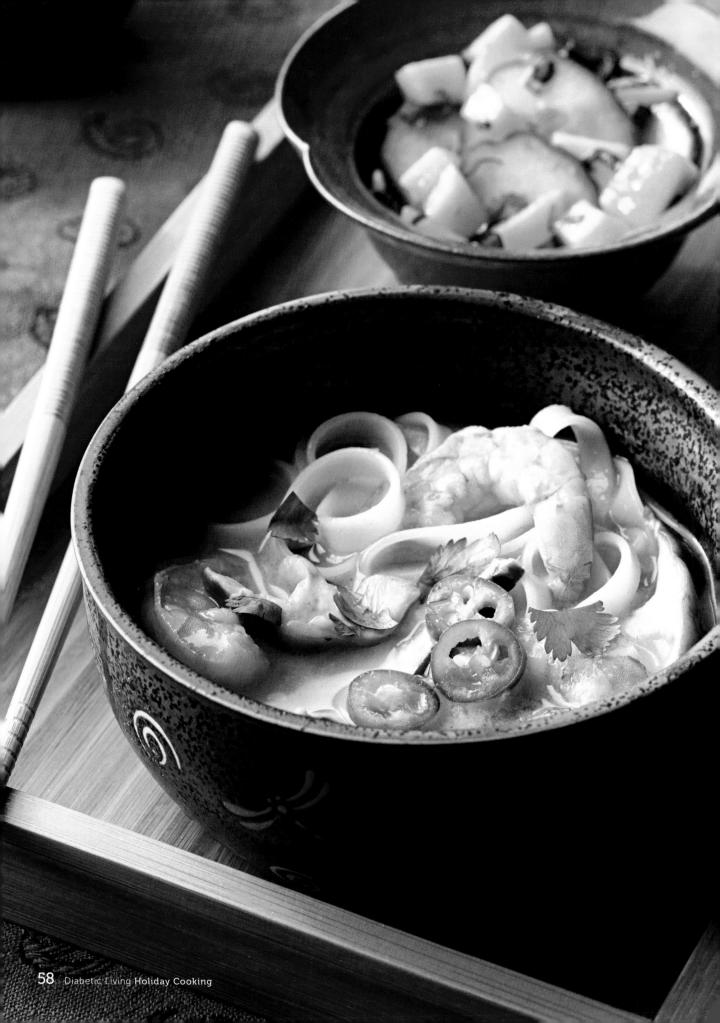

Thai Shrimp Coconut Soup with Mango Cucumber Salad

Shiitake mushroom stems are tough and woody and should not be eaten. Cut off the stems and discard them before slicing the caps.

SERVINGS 6 (1$\frac{1}{3}$ cups soup and about $\frac{1}{3}$ cup salad each)
CARB. PER SERVING 32 g or 31 g
START TO FINISH 55 minutes

- 1 pound fresh or frozen medium shrimp in shells
- 3 ounces rice noodles
- 2 teaspoons canola oil
- $\frac{1}{4}$ cup finely chopped onion
- 2 tablespoons finely chopped fresh lemongrass
- 4 cloves garlic, minced
- 1 teaspoon grated fresh ginger
- 1 teaspoon red curry paste
- 2$\frac{3}{4}$ cups unsalted chicken stock
- 1$\frac{1}{4}$ cups unsweetened light coconut milk
- 2 tablespoons packed brown sugar*
- 1 tablespoon fish sauce
- 4 ounces fresh stemmed shiitake and/or oyster mushrooms, sliced
- 2 tablespoons lime juice
- $\frac{1}{4}$ cup fresh cilantro leaves (optional)
- 1 fresh serrano chile pepper, very thinly sliced** (optional)
- 1 recipe Mango Cucumber Salad

PER SERVING: 270 cal., 7 g total fat (3 g sat. fat), 122 mg chol., 548 mg sodium, 32 g carb. (2 g fiber, 15 g sugars), 20 g pro. Exchanges: 1 vegetable, 0.5 fruit, 1.5 starch, 2 lean meat, 0.5 fat.

PER SERVING WITH SUBSTITUTE: Same as above, except 267 cal., 31 g carb.

1 | Thaw shrimp, if frozen. Peel and devein shrimp. Rinse shrimp; pat dry with paper towels. Set aside. Cook rice noodles according to package directions. Drain; set aside.

2 | In a 4-quart Dutch oven heat oil over medium heat. Add onion and lemongrass; cook and stir for 3 minutes. Add garlic, ginger, and red curry paste. Cook and stir about 1 minute more or until fragrant.

3 | Stir chicken stock, coconut milk, brown sugar, and fish sauce into onion mixture. Bring to boiling; reduce heat. Simmer, uncovered, for 5 minutes. Stir in shrimp and mushrooms. Simmer for 2 to 3 minutes more or until shrimp are opaque. Stir in lime juice.

4 | To serve, divide rice noodles among six soup bowls. Ladle soup over noodles. If desired, garnish with cilantro and sliced chile pepper. Serve with Mango Cucumber Salad.

MANGO CUCUMBER SALAD: For dressing, in a screw-top jar combine 2 tablespoons rice vinegar, 2 tablespoons snipped fresh basil, 1 tablespoon canola oil, 1 teaspoon brown sugar,* $\frac{1}{2}$ teaspoon Asian chili sauce (Sriracha sauce), and $\frac{1}{8}$ teaspoon salt. Cover and shake well. Halve 2 medium mangoes; remove seeds, peel, and chop. In a medium bowl combine mangoes and 1 cup sliced, seeded cucumber. Drizzle with dressing. Serve immediately or cover and chill for up to 2 hours.

*SUGAR SUBSTITUTES: We do not recommend using a sugar substitute for the soup. Choose from Sugar Twin Brown or Sweet'N Low Brown for the Mango Cucumber Salad. Follow package directions to use product amount equivalent to 1 teaspoon brown sugar.

**TEST KITCHEN TIP: Because chile peppers contain volatile oils that can burn your skin and eyes, avoid direct contact with them as much as possible. When working with chile peppers, wear plastic or rubber gloves. If your bare hands do touch the peppers, wash your hands and nails well with soap and warm water.

Roasted Carrot Soup

For easy cleanup, line the baking pan with foil before adding the vegetables. For even roasting, be sure to arrange the vegetables in a single layer.

SERVINGS 4 (1¼ cups each)
CARB. PER SERVING 21 g
PREP 20 minutes **BAKE** 50 minutes

1½ pounds carrots, peeled and cut into 2- to 3-inch pieces

1 onion, peeled and quartered

3 cloves garlic, unpeeled

1 1-inch piece fresh ginger, peeled and sliced

1 tablespoon olive oil

2 cups unsweetened almond milk

1 cup low-sodium chicken broth

1 teaspoon coarsely ground black pepper

1 cup water

Shredded carrot (optional)

Fresh basil leaves (optional)

1 Preheat oven to 400°F. In a large bowl combine carrot pieces, onion, garlic, and ginger. Drizzle with oil; toss to coat. Arrange vegetables in a single layer in a 15×10×1-inch baking pan. Bake for 50 to 60 minutes or until carrots are very tender. Cool slightly.

2 Squeeze garlic cloves from their skins into a food processor or blender. Add roasted carrots, onion, and ginger; cover and process or blend with several on/off turns until the vegetables are chopped. Add almond milk, broth, and pepper. Cover and process or blend until smooth.

3 Transfer to a medium saucepan. Stir in the water. Cook and stir until heated through. Ladle into four soup bowls. If desired, garnish with shredded carrot and basil leaves.

QUICK TIP

If using a blender, cover the hole in the middle of the lid with a towel so the bright orange mixture does not splatter out.

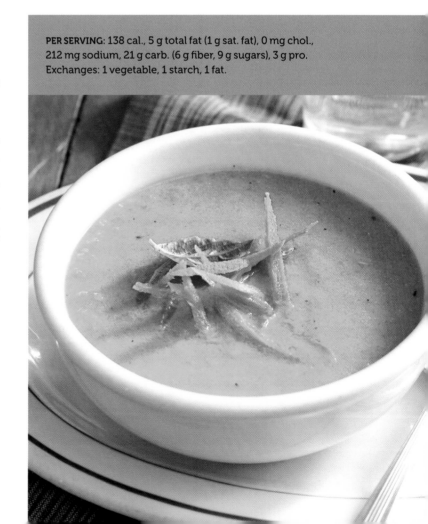

PER SERVING: 138 cal., 5 g total fat (1 g sat. fat), 0 mg chol., 212 mg sodium, 21 g carb. (6 g fiber, 9 g sugars), 3 g pro. Exchanges: 1 vegetable, 1 starch, 1 fat.

Pumpkin Soup with Lentils

Golden hues and sweetly spiced flavors shine through in this hearty meatless soup. The earthy lentils provide good-for-you protein.

SERVINGS 4 (1¹/₂ cups each)
CARB. PER SERVING 29 g
PREP 20 minutes   COOK 25 minutes

- 1 small sweet onion, cut into wedges
- 1 yellow sweet pepper, seeded and sliced
- ¹/₂ cup lentils, rinsed and well drained
- 1 tablespoon olive oil
- 2 teaspoons grated fresh ginger
- 1 teaspoon curry powder
- 1 teaspoon ground cumin
- 3¹/₄ cups reduced-sodium chicken broth
- 1 15-ounce can pumpkin
- ¹/₈ teaspoon salt
- ¹/₈ teaspoon black pepper
- Freshly grated nutmeg (optional)
- Snipped fresh Italian (flat-leaf) parsley (optional)

PER SERVING: 187 cal., 4 g total fat (1 g sat. fat), 0 mg chol., 533 mg sodium, 29 g carb. (11 g fiber, 6 g sugars), 11 g pro. Exchanges: 1 vegetable, 1.5 starch, 0.5 lean meat, 0.5 fat.

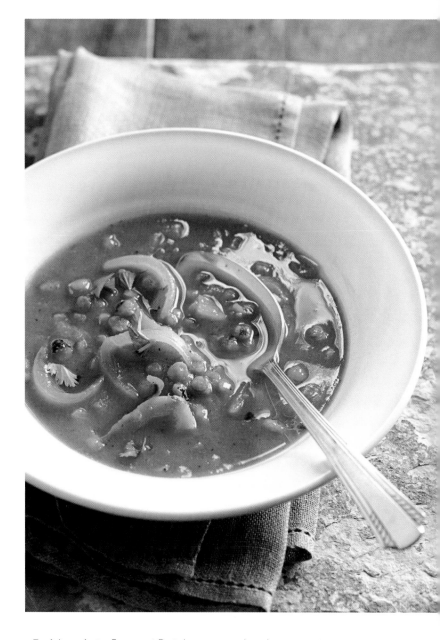

1 In a 4- to 5- quart Dutch oven cook onion, sweet pepper, and lentils in hot oil over medium-high heat for 2 minutes. Whisk in ginger, curry powder, cumin, broth, and pumpkin. Bring to boiling; reduce heat to medium-low. Simmer, covered, for 25 minutes or until lentils are tender, stirring occasionally. Season with the salt and black pepper.

2 Ladle into four soup bowls and, if desired, sprinkle with grated nutmeg and parsley.

Greek Lemony Rice Soup with Pita Salad

The blended tofu and egg mixture helps create a consistency and appearance similar to a cream-base soup. And it's lower in fat.

SERVINGS 6 (1$^{1}/_{3}$ cups soup and $^{1}/_{2}$ cup salad each)
CARB. PER SERVING 27 g
PREP 40 minutes COOK 20 minutes

- 2 bone-in chicken breast halves (about 1$^{1}/_{2}$ pounds total)
- $^{1}/_{8}$ teaspoon salt
- $^{1}/_{8}$ teaspoon black pepper
- 2 teaspoons butter
- $^{1}/_{2}$ cup chopped onion (1 medium)
- 4 cups unsalted chicken stock
- 8 ounces soft silken-style tofu (fresh bean curd)
- 2 eggs
- $^{1}/_{4}$ cup lemon juice
- $^{1}/_{4}$ teaspoon salt
- 2 cups cooked brown rice
- 2 tablespoons slivered green onions
- Shredded lemon or lime peel (optional)
- Freshly ground black pepper (optional)
- 1 recipe Pita Salad

1 Remove and discard skin from chicken breasts. Sprinkle chicken with the $^{1}/_{8}$ teaspoon salt and the $^{1}/_{8}$ teaspoon pepper. In a 4-quart Dutch oven melt butter over medium heat. Add chicken; cook for 3 minutes, turning once. Add onion; cook for 3 minutes more. Add chicken stock. Bring to boiling; reduce heat. Simmer, covered, for 20 to 30 minutes or until chicken is no longer pink (170°F). Transfer chicken to a cutting board; reserve cooking liquid. When chicken is cool enough to handle, remove and discard bones. Cut chicken into bite-size pieces; set aside.

2 In a blender or food processor combine tofu, eggs, lemon juice, and the $^{1}/_{4}$ teaspoon salt. Cover and blend or process until smooth. Gradually stir about 1 cup of the reserved hot cooking liquid into the tofu mixture. Gradually add tofu mixture to the remaining cooking liquid in the Dutch oven, whisking constantly. Cook and stir for 1 to 2 minutes or until an instant-read thermometer inserted into center of soup registers 160°F and the mixture coats the back of a clean metal spoon (do not boil).

3 Remove from heat. Stir in cooked rice and cut-up chicken. Ladle into six soup bowls. Top with green onions. If desired, sprinkle with shredded lemon peel and/or freshly ground black pepper. Serve with Pita Salad.

PITA SALAD: For dressing, in a screw-top jar combine 2 tablespoons red wine vinegar, 1 tablespoon olive oil, 1 tablespoon snipped fresh oregano, and $^{1}/_{4}$ teaspoon black pepper. Cover and shake well to combine; set aside. Break 2 ounces plain pita chips into bite-size pieces (about 1$^{1}/_{4}$ cups broken). In large bowl combine pita chip pieces, 1 cup chopped tomatoes, $^{1}/_{2}$ cup chopped cucumber, $^{1}/_{4}$ cup chopped pitted Kalamata olives, and $^{1}/_{4}$ cup crumbled reduced-fat feta cheese. Drizzle with dressing; toss gently to coat. Serve immediately.

27 grams pro.

PER SERVING: 328 cal., 12 g total fat (3 g sat. fat), 114 mg chol., 603 mg sodium, 27 g carb. (3 g fiber, 2 g sugars), 27 g pro. Exchanges: 0.5 vegetable, 1.5 starch, 3 lean meat, 1 fat.

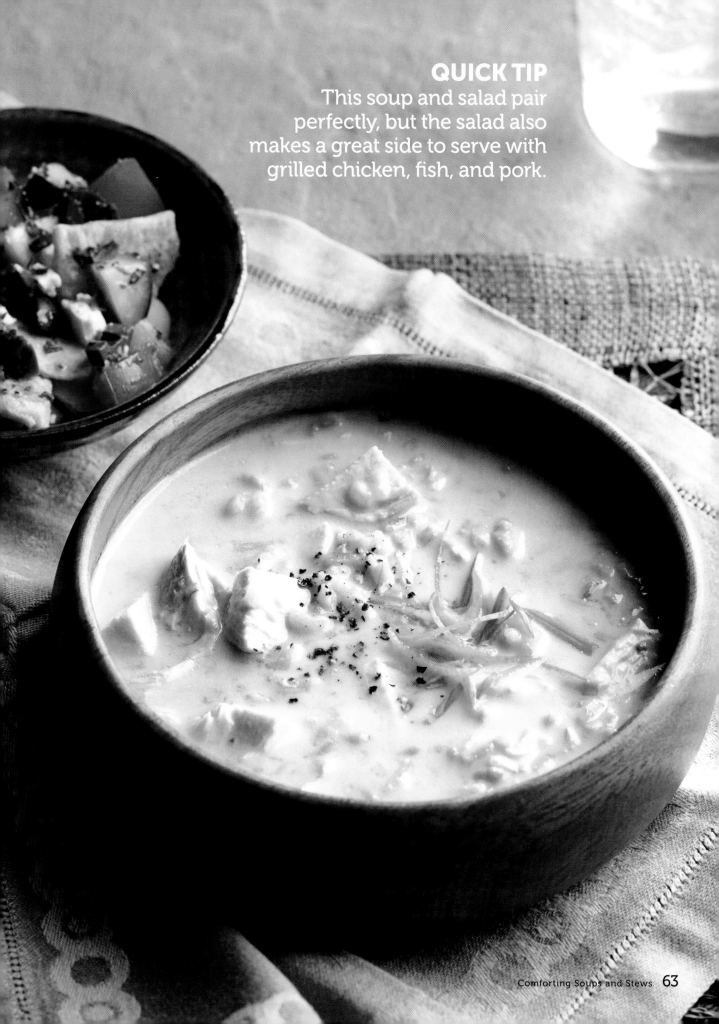

QUICK TIP
This soup and salad pair perfectly, but the salad also makes a great side to serve with grilled chicken, fish, and pork.

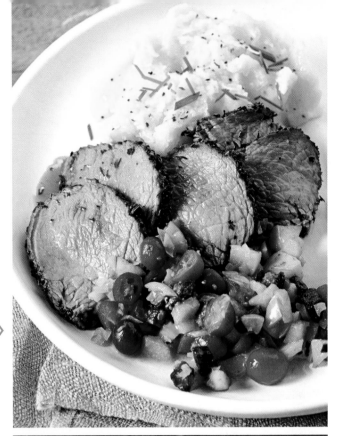

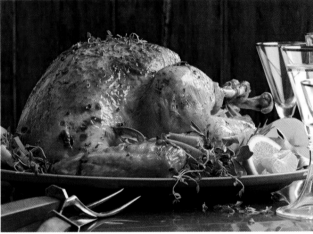

4

main-dish
masterpieces

It's quite simple during the holiday season to gravitate toward

healthful eating if there are eye-appealing, palate-pleasing dishes

on the table. Take your pick from these festive entrées—each is

lightened up to deliver a package of calorie, carbohydrate, and

fat numbers that will keep your meal plan in check.

Beef Pot Roast and Polenta with Shiitake Cream Sauce

For lump-free polenta, use a wire whisk to stir the mixture while bringing it to a boil.

SERVINGS 8 (3 ounces cooked beef, $^1/_3$ cup vegetables, 2 pieces polenta, and $^1/_4$ cup sauce each)
CARB. PER SERVING 23 g
PREP 30 minutes CHILL 4 hours
BAKE 2 hours 15 minutes
COOK 5 minutes

1 recipe Polenta (see recipe, *page 67*)

1 2- to 2$^1/_2$-pound boneless beef chuck pot roast

6 cloves garlic, minced

1 tablespoon snipped fresh rosemary or 1 teaspoon dried rosemary, finely crushed

1 tablespoon snipped fresh oregano or 1 teaspoon dried oregano, finely crushed

$^1/_2$ teaspoon salt

$^1/_4$ teaspoon black pepper

4 teaspoons canola oil

8 medium carrots, cut into 2-inch pieces

1 large onion, cut into thin wedges

$^3/_4$ cup 50 percent-less-sodium beef broth

1 0.75-ounce package dried shiitake mushrooms

$^3/_4$ cup boiling water

$^3/_4$ cup fat-free half-and-half

3 tablespoons flour

$^1/_8$ teaspoon salt

4 teaspoons canola oil

PER SERVING: 305 cal., 10 g total fat (2 g sat. fat), 75 mg chol., 448 mg sodium, 23 g carb. (3 g fiber, 5 g sugars), 29 g pro. Exchanges: 1.5 vegetable, 1 starch, 3 lean meat, 1 fat.

1 Prepare Polenta; cover and chill for at least 4 hours or overnight.

2 Preheat oven to 350°F. Trim fat from beef. Cut beef into 4- to 5-inch pieces. Rub beef pieces evenly with garlic. In a small bowl combine rosemary, oregano, $^1/_2$ teaspoon salt, and pepper. Sprinkle evenly over all sides of beef pieces, rubbing in with your fingers.

3 In a 6- to 8-quart Dutch oven heat 4 teaspoons oil over medium heat. Add half of the beef pieces. Cook until browned, turning to brown all sides. Transfer to a plate; set aside. Repeat with remaining beef pieces and remove from the pan. Add carrot pieces and onion wedges to the same pan. Place beef pieces on top of vegetables in pan. Add broth to pan. Bring to boiling. Cover and bake for 2$^1/_4$ to 2$^1/_2$ hours or until beef is tender.

4 In a small bowl combine mushroom caps and the boiling water; cover and let stand for 20 minutes. Strain mushrooms through a fine-mesh sieve, reserving the soaking liquid. Rinse the mushrooms well. Chop the mushrooms. Set mushrooms and soaking liquid aside.

5 Transfer beef and vegetables to an ovenproof serving platter; cover the platter with foil. Turn off the oven and set the platter in the oven to keep warm. Pour juices from the pan into a 2-cup glass measure. If necessary, discard enough so you are left with $^3/_4$ cup or add enough reduced-sodium beef broth or water to equal $^3/_4$ cup. Pour back into the Dutch oven. Add mushrooms and soaking liquid. In a small bowl whisk together fat-free half-and-half, flour, and $^1/_8$ teaspoon salt until smooth. Add to mushroom mixture. Cook and stir until cream sauce is thickened and bubbly; cook and stir for 1 minute more. Cover and keep warm over very low heat.

6 To finish polenta, lift polenta out of pan and cut into 16 squares. In a large nonstick skillet heat 4 teaspoons oil over medium heat. Add polenta squares. Cook for 3 to 5 minutes or until heated through and lightly browned, turning once halfway through cooking.

7 Divide polenta squares among eight serving plates. Spoon cream sauce evenly over polenta. Cut beef into serving-size portions; add beef and vegetables to serving plates.

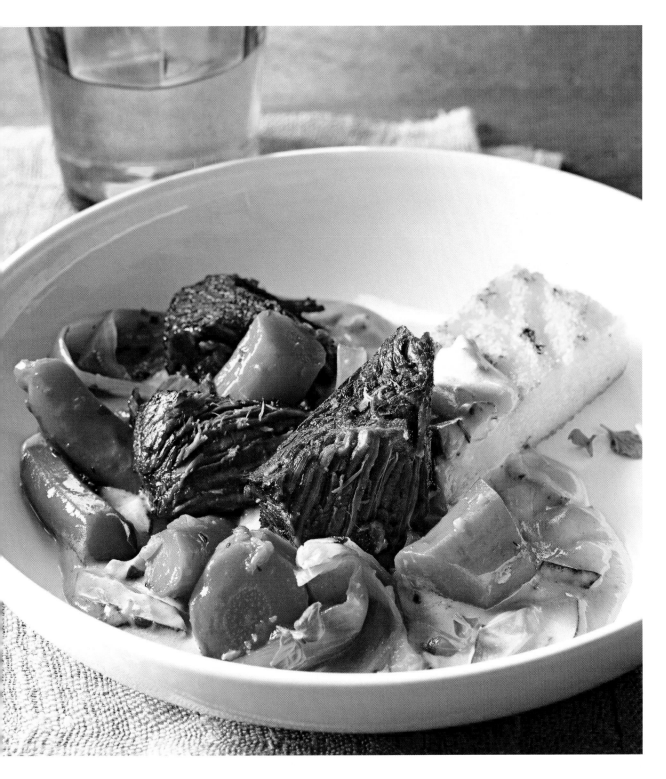

POLENTA: Line an 8×8×2-inch baking pan with foil; set aside. In a medium saucepan combine 2¾ cups cold water, ¾ cup yellow cornmeal, and ¼ teaspoon salt. Bring to boiling, whisking constantly. Reduce heat; simmer, uncovered, about 10 minutes or until very thick, stirring frequently. Pour cooked polenta into prepared pan. Cool for 10 minutes. Cover and chill at least 4 hours or overnight. (If desired, omit the 2¾ cups water, the cornmeal, and ¼ teaspoon salt. Use one 16-ounce tube refrigerated cooked polenta. Cut the tube of polenta crosswise into eight slices and cook as directed in Step 6.)

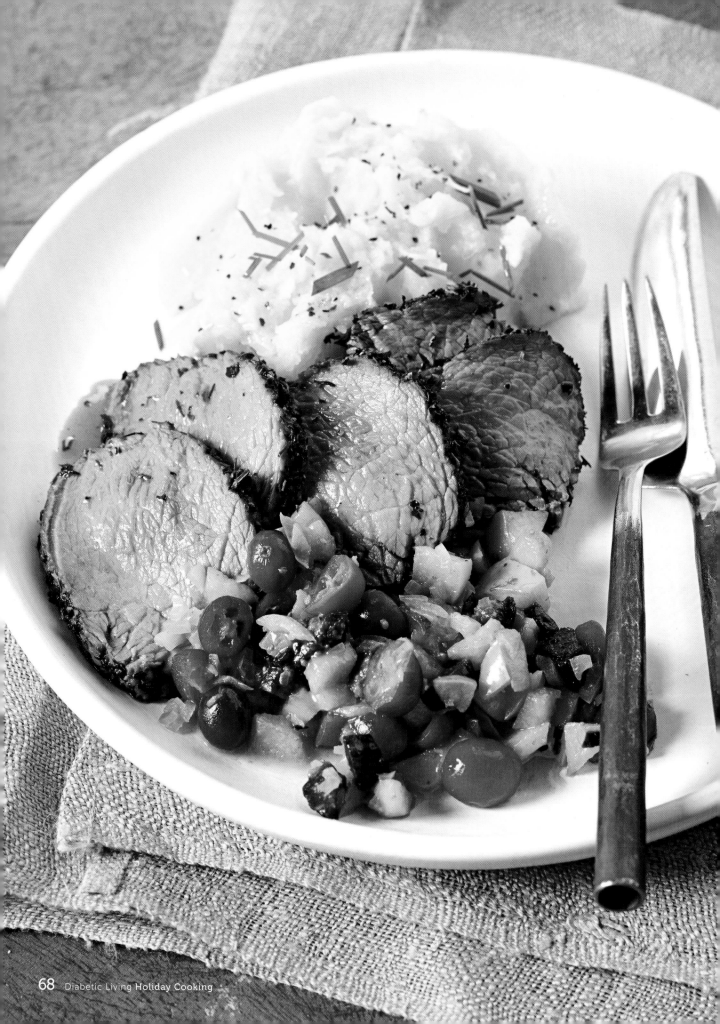

Roast Beef with Fig-Cranberry Chutney and Horseradish Potatoes

Shoulder petite tenders are typically very lean and free of fat. If there is any visible fat on the outside, give it a trim.

SERVINGS 6 (3 ounces cooked beef, $^2/_3$ cup potatoes, and 2 tablespoons chutney each)
CARB. PER SERVING 34 g
PREP 45 minutes ROAST 25 minutes COOK 25 minutes STAND 5 minutes

2 10-ounce beef shoulder petite tenders

1 tablespoon herbes de Provence, crushed

$^1/_2$ teaspoon salt

$^1/_4$ teaspoon black pepper

1 pound Yukon gold or russet potatoes, peeled and cut into 2-inch pieces

3 medium parsnips, peeled and cut into 2-inch pieces (about 1 pound)

$^1/_2$ cup fat-free milk, warmed

2 tablespoons light butter

2 to 3 teaspoons prepared horseradish

$^1/_2$ teaspoon salt

$^1/_8$ teaspoon black pepper

2 tablespoons thinly sliced fresh chives (optional)

1 recipe Fig-Cranberry Chutney

PER SERVING: 304 cal., 9 g total fat (4 g sat. fat), 61 mg chol., 539 mg sodium, 34 g carb. (6 g fiber, 10 g sugars), 23 g pro. Exchanges: 0.5 fruit, 1.5 starch, 3 lean meat, 0.5 fat.

1 Preheat oven to 425°F. Sprinkle all sides of tenders evenly with herbes de Provence, $^1/_2$ teaspoon salt, and $^1/_4$ teaspoon pepper, rubbing in with your fingers. Place petite tenders on a rack in a shallow roasting pan.

2 Roast, uncovered, for 25 to 30 minutes or until an instant-read thermometer inserted in centers of tenders registers 145°F for medium rare or 160°F for medium. Cover meat with foil; let stand for 5 minutes before serving.

3 While meat is roasting, in a 4- to 5-quart Dutch oven cook potatoes and parsnips, covered, in enough boiling water to cover for 25 to 30 minutes or until vegetables are very tender. Drain and return to the Dutch oven.

4 Mash with a potato masher or beat with an electric mixer on medium speed until mashed. Add milk, 2 tablespoons light butter, horseradish, $^1/_2$ teaspoon salt, and $^1/_8$ teaspoon pepper. Mash or beat until smooth. If desired, stir in chives just before serving. To serve, thinly slice beef crosswise. Divide beef evenly among six serving plates. Spoon chutney over meat. Spoon mashed potatoes evenly onto each plate.

FIG-CRANBERRY CHUTNEY: In a small saucepan cook $^1/_4$ cup finely chopped shallots in 2 teaspoons light butter over medium heat for 3 to 4 minutes or until tender, stirring occasionally. Peel, core, and chop 1 small cooking apple. Add to saucepan with shallots and cook, covered, over medium heat for 3 minutes, stirring occasionally. Add $^1/_2$ cup fresh cranberries; $^1/_4$ cup chopped, stemmed dried Mission figs; $^1/_4$ cup water; and dash salt. Bring to boiling; reduce heat. Simmer, covered, for 4 to 6 minutes or until cranberry skins have popped and figs are tender, stirring occasionally. Remove from the heat. Stir in 1 teaspoon cider vinegar just before serving.

Sirloin Steak with Deep Red Wine Reduction

When selecting a wine for cooking, pick one that is good for drinking. If a wine is not good enough to drink, it's not good enough to cook with.

SERVINGS 4 (3 ounces cooked steak and 1 tablespoon sauce each)
CARB. PER SERVING 4 g
PREP 15 minutes MARINATE 8 hours
COOK 10 minutes STAND 3 minutes

½ cup dry red wine

2 tablespoons balsamic vinegar

1 tablespoon reduced-sodium soy sauce

2 teaspoons instant coffee granules

2 teaspoons Worcestershire sauce

½ teaspoon coarsely ground black pepper

1 pound boneless beef sirloin steak, trimmed and cut about ¾ inch thick

⅛ teaspoon salt

Nonstick cooking spray

Steamed sliced zucchini and/or yellow summer squash (optional)

Snipped fresh oregano (optional)

PER SERVING: 162 cal., 5 g total fat (2 g sat. fat), 61 mg chol., 297 mg sodium, 4 g carb. (0 g fiber, 1 g sugars), 20 g pro. Exchanges: 0.5 fruit, 3 lean meat.

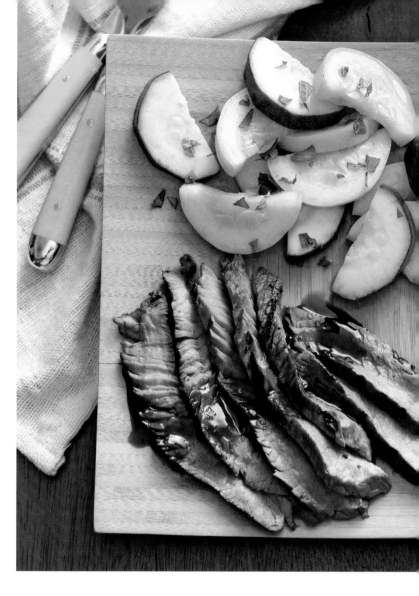

1 | In a small bowl combine wine, vinegar, soy sauce, coffee granules, Worcestershire sauce, and pepper. Place the steak in a large resealable plastic bag set in a shallow dish. Pour ¼ cup of the wine mixture over the steak. Seal bag; turn to coat steak. Marinate in the refrigerator for 8 to 24 hours, turning occasionally. Stir the salt into the remaining wine mixture; cover and chill until needed.

2 | Lightly coat a grill pan with cooking spray. Heat over medium-high heat. Drain steak, discarding marinade. Cook steak on hot grill pan for 10 to 12 minutes or until desired doneness (145°F for medium rare), turning once halfway through cooking time. Transfer steak to a cutting board. Let stand for 3 minutes; thinly slice steak.

3 | Meanwhile, in a small saucepan heat the reserved wine mixture to boiling over medium-high heat. Boil, uncovered, for 2 to 3 minutes or until mixture is reduced to ¼ cup. Spoon wine mixture over sliced steak. If desired, serve steak with zucchini sprinkled with oregano.

Petite Tenderloin with Chipotle Sweet Potatoes

Filet mignon are steaks cut from the small end of the beef tenderloin. Request that the butcher cut two 4-ounce, 1-inch-thick portions.

SERVINGS 2 (4 ounces cooked steak, $^1/_2$ cup sweet potatoes, and 2 tablespoons sauce each)
CARB. PER SERVING 24 g
PREP 20 minutes COOK 15 minutes

- 1 8-ounce sweet potato, peeled and cubed
- 1 tablespoon light butter
- 1 to 2 teaspoons finely chopped canned chipotle chile peppers in adobo sauce*
- 2 4-ounce beef filet mignon steaks, about 1 inch thick
- $1^1/_2$ teaspoons olive oil
- 1 recipe Cilantro Chimichurri

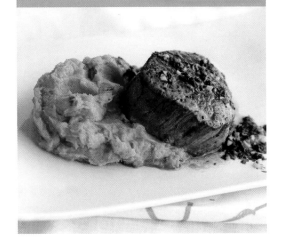

PER SERVING: 315 cal., 14 g total fat (4 g sat. fat), 59 mg chol., 313 mg sodium, 24 g carb. (4 g fiber, 5 g sugars), 22 g pro. Exchanges: 1.5 starch, 3 lean meat, 1.5 fat.

1 In a covered medium saucepan cook sweet potato in boiling water to cover for 15 to 20 minutes or until tender; drain well. Mash with a potato masher or beat with an electric mixer on low speed until smooth. Stir in butter and chile peppers until mixed.

2 Meanwhile, trim fat from steaks. Heat oil a large skillet over medium heat. Cook steaks in skillet for 10 to 13 minutes or until medium rare (145°F), turning once. Transfer steaks to a platter. Cover with foil; let stand for 5 minutes while preparing chimichurri.

3 Serve steak with sweet potatoes. Top with the Cilantro Chimichurri.

CILANTRO CHIMICHURRI: In a small bowl stir together $^1/_2$ cup finely snipped fresh cilantro leaves; 2 teaspoons red wine vinegar; 1 teaspoon olive oil; 1 clove garlic, minced; and $^1/_8$ teaspoon salt. Spoon onto steaks and sweet potatoes.

*TEST KITCHEN TIP: Because chile peppers contain volatile oils that can burn your skin and eyes, avoid direct contact with them as much as possible. When working with chile peppers, wear plastic or rubber gloves. If your bare hands do touch the peppers, wash your hands and nails well with soap and warm water.

QUICK TIP
Let steaks stand for 5 minutes after cooking so the juices redistribute throughout the tender meat.

Brined Classic Roast Turkey

Stuffing the turkey with aromatics—fruits, vegetables, and herbs—helps to infuse the meat with hints of delicious flavors during roasting.

SERVINGS 10 (6 ounces turkey)
CARB. PER SERVING 1 g
PREP 15 minutes CHILL 12 hours
ROAST 2 hours 45 minutes
STAND 15 minutes

- 3 quarts water
- 2 quarts apple cider
- 1 cup kosher salt
- 2/3 cup packed brown sugar*
- 2 oranges, sliced
- 2 bay leaves
- 2 tablespoons crystallized ginger
- 1 tablespoon whole black peppercorns
- 2 teaspoons whole allspice
- 12 cups ice
- 1 10- to 12-pound turkey
- 1 recipe Turkey Aromatics
- 2 teaspoons vegetable oil
- 1/4 teaspoon salt
- 1/8 teaspoon black pepper
- 1 recipe Turkey Gravy (optional) (see recipe, *page 73*)

PER SERVING: 302 cal., 8 g total fat
(2 g sat. fat), 183 mg chol.,
558 mg sodium, 1 g carb. (0 g fiber,
1 g sugars), 53 g pro.
Exchanges: 7 lean meat.

1 For the brine, in a 16-quart stockpot combine the water, apple cider, kosher salt, brown sugar, orange slices, bay leaves, crystallized ginger, peppercorns, and allspice. Cover; heat over high heat until brine is steaming, stirring occasionally to dissolve salt and brown sugar. Remove from heat. Add the ice; let stand until ice melts and brine is cool. Remove neck and giblets from turkey; reserve for another use or discard. Rinse the turkey body cavity. Place turkey in stockpot with cooled brine. Weight down turkey with several plates. Cover; chill for 12 to 16 hours.

2 Preheat oven to 325°F. Remove turkey from brine, draining excess brine from cavity; discard brine. Pat turkey dry with paper towels. Insert Turkey Aromatics loosely into body cavity. Skewer neck skin to back. Tuck drumstick ends under band of skin across the tail if present or tie drumsticks securely to the tail using 100-percent-cotton kitchen string. Twist wing tips under back.

3 Place turkey, breast side up, on a rack in a shallow roasting pan. Brush with the oil and sprinkle with the salt and pepper. Insert an oven-going meat thermometer into the center of an inside thigh muscle (the thermometer should not touch bone). Cover turkey loosely with foil.

4 Roast turkey for 2¼ hours. Remove foil; cut band of skin or string between drumsticks so thighs cook evenly. Roast for 30 to 45 minutes more or until the meat thermometer registers at least 175°F when thermometer is inserted in the thigh. (The juices should run clear and drumsticks should move easily in their sockets.) Remove turkey from oven. Cover with foil; let stand for 15 to 20 minutes before carving. Transfer turkey to a cutting board; remove and discard Turkey Aromatics. Remove skin and discard. Carve turkey. If desired, serve with Turkey Gravy and garnish with *fresh fruit* and *fresh herbs*.

TURKEY AROMATICS: Insert 1 medium orange, cut into wedges (leave peel on); 1 medium apple, cored and cut into wedges; 1 medium onion, cut into wedges; 1 small bulb garlic, top and bottom cut off to expose cloves; and 3 sprigs fresh sage, thyme, and/or rosemary into the turkey cavity.

*SUGAR SUBSTITUTE: We do not recommend using a sugar substitute for this recipe.

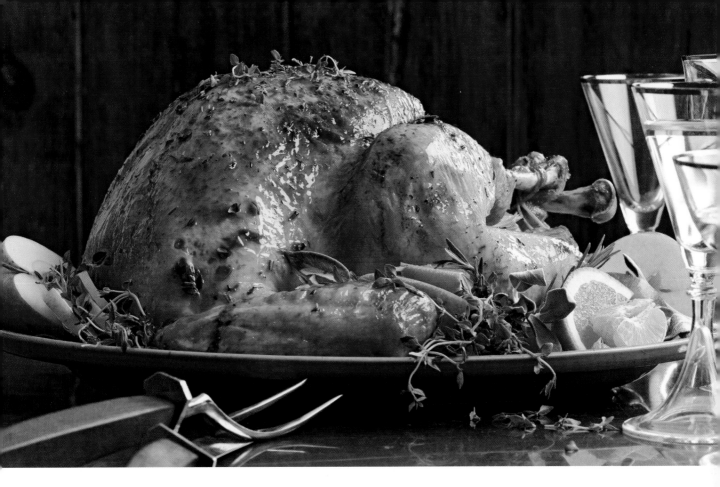

Turkey Gravy

Straining the gravy through a fine-mesh sieve will ensure that any small lumps don't make it into the gravy bowl.

SERVINGS 8 ($^1/_4$ cup each)
CARB. PER SERVING 3 g
START TO FINISH 15 minutes

Reduced-sodium chicken broth

Pan drippings from roasted turkey

Melted butter (optional)

$^1/_4$ cup flour

$^1/_4$ teaspoon salt

$^1/_8$ teaspoon black pepper

PER SERVING: 76 cal., 6 g total fat
(2 g sat. fat), 7 mg chol.,
211 mg sodium, 3 g carb. (0 g fiber,
0 g sugars), 1 g pro. Exchanges: 1 fat.

1 | Stir 1 cup chicken broth into pan drippings from roasted turkey in roasting pan, scraping up any browned bits from bottom of pan. Pour drippings into a 2-cup glass measuring cup. Skim and reserve fat from drippings. If necessary, add enough melted butter to the reserved fat to make $^1/_4$ cup. Add enough additional broth to the drippings in the measuring cup to make 2 cups total liquid.

2 | Pour the $^1/_4$ cup fat into a medium saucepan (discard any remaining fat). Stir in flour. Add broth mixture all at once to saucepan, stirring until smooth. Cook and stir over medium heat until thickened and bubbly. Cook and stir for 1 minute more. Stir in the salt and pepper. To serve, strain gravy into a serving bowl.

MAKE-AHEAD DIRECTIONS: Prepare gravy and place in an airtight container; cover. Store gravy in the refrigerator for up to 24 hours. To serve, in a small saucepan reheat gravy over medium-low heat until bubbling. If gravy is too thick, add additional chicken broth until desired consistency.

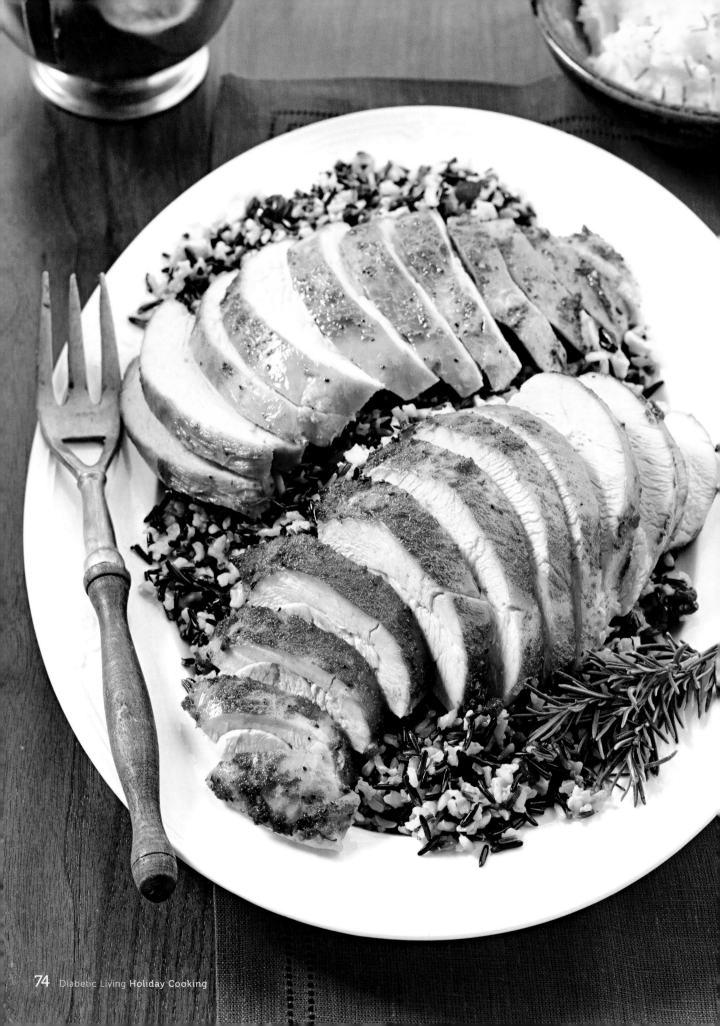

Honey-Lemon Glazed Turkey with Fruited Wild Rice

For beautiful slices, on each side of the breast cut along the bone to remove the meat in one piece, then cut the meat into slices.

SERVINGS 12 (3 ounces turkey and $^1/_3$ cup rice each)
CARB. PER SERVING 25 g
PREP 30 minutes   COOK 45 minutes   ROAST 2 hours 20 minutes   STAND 15 minutes

- 1   5- to 6-pound whole turkey breast on the bone
- 1   tablespoon paprika
- 1   teaspoon ground ginger
- $^1/_2$ teaspoon salt
- $^1/_2$ teaspoon black pepper
- $^1/_4$ teaspoon ground nutmeg
- $^1/_8$ teaspoon ground saffron
- 2   tablespoons lemon juice
- 2   tablespoons honey
- 1   recipe Fruited Wild Rice

PER SERVING: 277 cal., 4 g total fat (1 g sat. fat), 74 mg chol., 279 mg sodium, 25 g carb. (2 g fiber, 7 g sugars), 34 g pro. Exchanges: 1.5 starch, 4 lean meat.

1 Preheat oven to 350°F. Line a shallow roasting pan with foil. Place turkey on a rack in the pan. Loosen skin from the breast meat by running your finger under the skin. In a small bowl combine paprika, ginger, salt, pepper, nutmeg, and saffron. Spoon mixture under the skin, rubbing it evenly onto the meat with your fingers.

2 Roast turkey, uncovered, for 1$^1/_2$ hours. Meanwhile, in a small saucepan stir together lemon juice and honey until well combined. Remove turkey from oven and place pan on a wire rack. Carefully lift off the skin of the turkey, cutting it off the meat as needed. With a knife, remove any rub mixture that may be on the skin and spread over turkey breast; discard skin. Using a thin, sharp knife, make 10 to 12 slits into the meat. Gently brush about half of the lemon juice mixture over the meat; reserve remaining mixture in saucepan.

3 Cover turkey loosely with foil. Roast for 20 to 30 minutes more or until an instant-read thermometer inserted into thickest part of the breast registers 170°F.

4 Place the saucepan with the remaining lemon mixture over medium heat. Bring just to boiling, stirring frequently. Remove from heat. When turkey is finished, brush the remaining lemon mixture over turkey. Let stand in the pan on a wire rack, covered, for 15 minutes before carving. Remove turkey meat from the bones. Slice turkey and arrange on a serving platter. Serve with Fruited Wild Rice.

FRUITED WILD RICE: While turkey is roasting, in a 4-quart Dutch oven cook 1 cup chopped onion (1 large) in 2 tablespoons hot canola oil over medium heat for 5 minutes, stirring occasionally. Stir in 4 cloves garlic, minced. Add two 14.5-ounce cans reduced-sodium chicken broth; 1 cup wild rice, rinsed and drained; $^1/_2$ cup uncooked brown rice; $^1/_2$ cup water; $^1/_4$ cup dried apples, snipped; and $^1/_4$ cup dried cherries, snipped. Bring to boiling; reduce heat. Simmer, covered, for 45 to 50 minutes or until rice is tender and liquid is absorbed. Remove from heat; stir in 1 to 1$^1/_2$ teaspoons snipped fresh rosemary.

Chorizo-Stuffed Turkey Tenderloins with Sweet Potatoes

Kitchen string is used to keep the turkey rolls intact while cooking. Use kitchen scissors to snip the strings; remove before slicing and serving.

SERVINGS 6 (5 ounces turkey and $^{1}/_{2}$ cup sweet potatoes each)
CARB. PER SERVING 18 g
PREP 40 minutes COOK 11 minutes
ROAST 30 minutes
STAND 5 minutes

- $^{3}/_{4}$ cup chopped red sweet pepper (1 medium)
- 1 cup chopped onion (1 medium)
- 4 ounces uncooked ground chorizo
- 2 cups coarsely chopped, trimmed Swiss chard
- 3 10- to 12-ounce turkey breast tenderloins
- 2 teaspoons dried oregano, crushed
- 1 teaspoon paprika
- $^{1}/_{4}$ teaspoon salt
- $^{1}/_{4}$ teaspoon black pepper
  Nonstick cooking spray
- 2 medium sweet potatoes (about 1$^{1}/_{4}$ pounds total), peeled, halved lengthwise, and cut crosswise into $^{1}/_{2}$-inch-thick slices
- 1 tablespoon olive oil
- 2 cloves garlic, thinly sliced
- $^{1}/_{4}$ teaspoon salt
- $^{1}/_{4}$ teaspoon black pepper

1 Preheat oven to 400°F. In a large skillet cook sweet pepper, onion, and chorizo over medium heat until chorizo is cooked through and vegetables are tender, stirring occasionally and breaking up meat as it cooks. Drain off fat. Add chard. Cook and stir for 1 minute more.

2 Place a turkey breast tenderloin on a cutting board. With a knife parallel to the cutting board, split in half to, but not through, the other side. Open like a book. Repeat with remaining tenderloins. Place a tenderloin between two sheets of plastic wrap. Using a meat mallet or rolling pin, pound the turkey to a uniform $^{1}/_{2}$-inch thickness. Repeat with the remaining tenderloins. Remove the plastic wrap; spread one-third of the stuffing onto each tenderloin, leaving a border around the edge. Starting with a long side, roll the tenderloin up into a log. Secure at 2-inch intervals with 100-percent-cotton kitchen string.

3 In a small bowl combine oregano, paprika, $^{1}/_{4}$ teaspoon salt, and $^{1}/_{4}$ teaspoon pepper. Sprinkle over the tenderloins to coat.

4 Coat a very large oven-going skillet with cooking spray; heat over medium heat. Add tenderloins to skillet. Cook for 5 minutes on one side until bottoms are browned. Turn tenderloins.

5 Place skillet in the oven and bake tenderloins, uncovered, for 10 minutes.

6 Meanwhile, line a 15×10×1-inch baking pan with foil; lightly coat foil with cooking spray. Set aside. In a medium bowl toss sweet potatoes with olive oil, garlic, $^{1}/_{4}$ teaspoon salt, and $^{1}/_{4}$ teaspoon pepper. Arrange sweet potatoes in a single layer in the prepared baking pan. Bake potatoes alongside the turkey for 20 to 25 minutes or until potatoes are lightly browned and tender, turning once, and the turkey is no longer pink (170°F). Cover turkey with foil and let stand for 5 minutes.

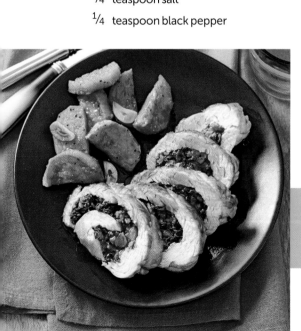

PER SERVING: 333 cal., 10 g total fat (3 g sat. fat), 104 mg chol., 561 mg sodium, 18 g carb. (3 g fiber, 4 g sugars), 41 g pro.
Exchanges: 0.5 vegetable, 1 starch, 5 lean meat, 0.5 fat.

Pork Tenderloin with Rich Onion-Cherry Chutney

Have all the chutney ingredients ready to roll so once the tenderloin goes in the oven to roast, you can start cooking the chutney.

SERVINGS 4 (3 ounces cooked pork and 3 tablespoons chutney each)
CARB. PER SERVING 18 g
PREP 25 minutes   ROAST 12 minutes
STAND 3 minutes

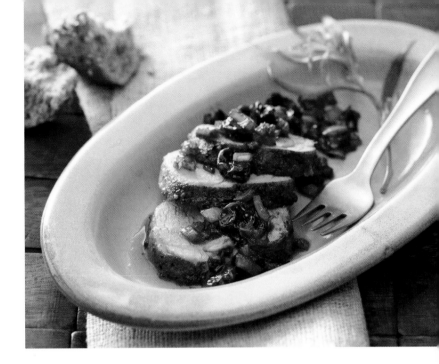

Nonstick cooking spray

- ½ teaspoon garlic powder
- ½ teaspoon ground allspice
- ½ teaspoon coarsely ground black pepper
- ⅛ teaspoon salt
- 1 1-pound pork tenderloin
- 4 teaspoons canola oil
- 1½ cups chopped onions (3 medium)
- ¼ cup dried cherries
- ¼ cup balsamic vinegar
- 1 teaspoon packed brown sugar*
- ⅛ teaspoon salt

Fresh tarragon sprigs (optional)

PER SERVING: 225 cal., 7 g total fat (1 g sat. fat), 70 mg chol., 200 mg sodium, 18 g carb. (2 g fiber, 12 g sugars), 24 g pro. Exchanges: 1 vegetable, 0.5 fruit, 3 lean meat, 0.5 fat.

PER SERVING WITH SUBSTITUTE: Same as above, except 10 g sugars.

1 Preheat oven to 425°F. Coat a 15×10×1-inch baking pan with cooking spray; set aside.

2 In a small bowl combine garlic powder, allspice, pepper, and ⅛ teaspoon salt. Sprinkle garlic powder mixture evenly over the tenderloin; rub in with your fingers.

3 In a very large nonstick skillet heat 1 teaspoon of the oil over medium-high heat; tilt skillet to coat bottom lightly with oil. Add tenderloin; cook about 6 minutes or until browned on both sides, turning once after 4 minutes of cooking. Place tenderloin on prepared baking pan. Roast, uncovered, for 12 to 15 minutes or until an instant-read thermometer inserted in center of tenderloin registers 145°F.

4 Meanwhile, for the chutney, in the same skillet heat the remaining 3 teaspoons oil over medium-high heat. Add onions. Cook and stir about 8 minutes or until golden brown, stirring to scrape up any browned bits from the bottom of the skillet. Add cherries, vinegar, and brown sugar. Cook and stir about 1 minute more or until most of the liquid has evaporated. Remove from heat. Stir in ⅛ teaspoon salt; set aside.

5 Place tenderloin on a cutting board; let stand for 3 minutes. Slice tenderloin. Serve tenderloin with the chutney. If desired, garnish with tarragon.

*SUGAR SUBSTITUTE: Choose Splenda Brown Sugar Blend. Follow package directions to use product amount equivalent to 1 teaspoon brown sugar.

Maple-Mustard Marinated Pork Loin with Parmesan-Crusted Vegetables

Finely crush the fennel seeds in a spice grinder. If you don't have one, try a mortar and pestle or use the bottom of a glass to crush seeds on a flat surface.

SERVINGS 8 (4 ounces cooked pork and ½ cup vegetables each)
CARB. PER SERVING 13 g
PREP 25 minutes   MARINATE 8 hours
ROAST 45 minutes   STAND 3 minutes

- 1   2- to 2½-pound boneless pork top loin roast (single loin)*
- ½   cup water
- ¼   cup pure maple syrup
- 2   tablespoons coarse-grain mustard
- 1   teaspoon salt
- 1   teaspoon black pepper
- 4   cloves garlic, minced
- 2   teaspoons fennel seeds, finely crushed
- 1   teaspoon ground coriander
- 2   medium fennel bulbs
- 3   cups Brussels sprouts, trimmed and halved
- 2   medium zucchini, trimmed, halved lengthwise, and cut crosswise into ½-inch-thick slices (2½ cups)
- 2   medium shallots, peeled and cut into thin wedges
- 2   tablespoons olive oil
- ¼   teaspoon salt
- ¼   teaspoon black pepper
- ⅓   cup finely shredded Parmesan cheese (½ ounce)
- ⅓   cup panko bread crumbs

PER SERVING: 249 cal., 9 g total fat (2 g sat. fat), 74 mg chol., 252 mg sodium, 13 g carb. (4 g fiber, 3 g sugars), 29 g pro. Exchanges: 2 vegetable, 3.5 lean meat, 0.5 fat.

1 | Trim fat from pork. Poke a thin sharp knife into the pork loin in eight to 10 different places. Place pork in a large resealable plastic bag set in a shallow dish. In a small bowl combine water, syrup, mustard, ½ teaspoon of the salt, and ½ teaspoon of the pepper. Pour over pork in bag. Seal bag; turn to coat pork. Marinate in the refrigerator for 8 to 24 hours, turning bag occasionally.

2 | Preheat oven to 400°F. Remove pork from marinade, discarding leftover marinade. Rub pork all over with the garlic. Sprinkle all over with fennel seeds, coriander, remaining ½ teaspoon salt, and remaining ½ teaspoon pepper. Place pork on a rack in a shallow roasting pan.

3 | Roast, uncovered, for 45 to 60 minutes or until an instant-read thermometer inserted into thickest part of the roast registers 145°F. Cover roast with foil. Let stand for 3 minutes before slicing.

4 | Meanwhile, trim upper stalks off the fennel bulbs and discard. Trim a thin slice off the base of each fennel bulb. Cut bulbs in half and cut out the cores. Thinly slice the bulbs. You should have about 3 cups. In a 15×10×1-inch baking pan combine sliced fennel, Brussels sprouts, zucchini, and shallots. Drizzle with oil and sprinkle with the ¼ teaspoon salt and pepper. Toss to coat.

5 | Roast, uncovered, in the oven with the pork for 15 to 20 minutes or until vegetables are just tender and starting to brown, stirring once halfway through roasting.

6 | In a small bowl combine cheese and bread crumbs. Sprinkle over vegetable mixture. Roast, uncovered, for 5 minutes more or until topping is browned. Thinly slice the pork and place on a large serving platter. Add vegetables to the platter. Serve warm.

*TEST KITCHEN TIP: Choose a pork roast that has not had any salt solution or marinade already added.

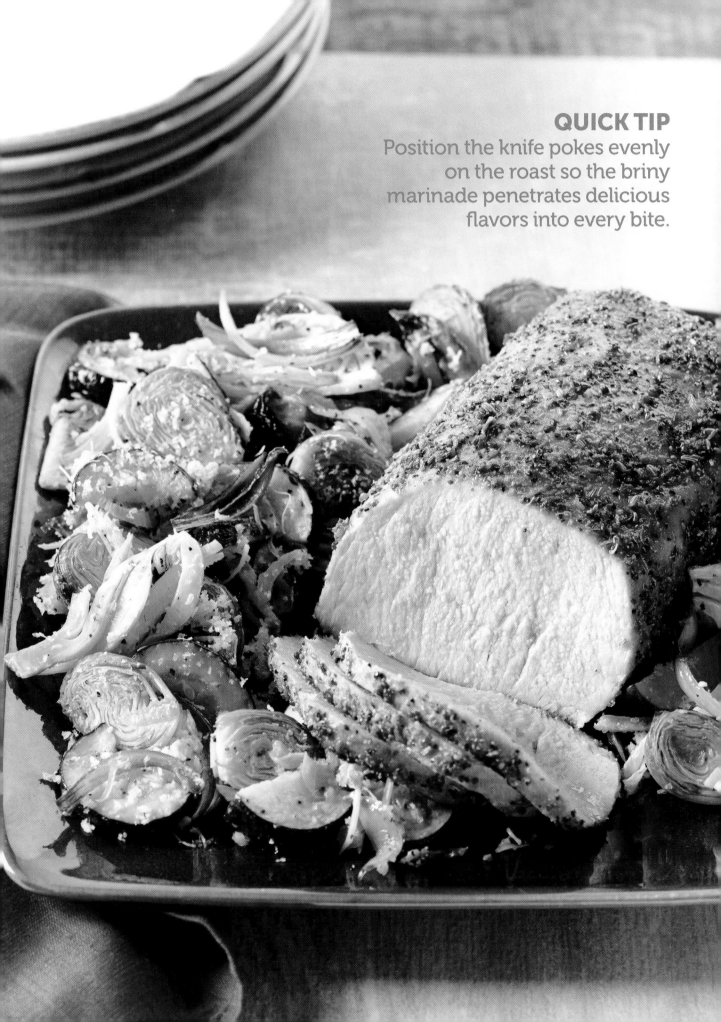

QUICK TIP
Position the knife pokes evenly on the roast so the briny marinade penetrates delicious flavors into every bite.

Sweet Orange Chicken over Kale

To remove the skin from a chicken thigh, use a paper towel to grip the skin on one side of the thigh, then pull it away from the meat.

SERVINGS 4 (1 chicken thigh and 1 cup kale mixture each)
CARB. PER SERVING 27 g
PREP 35 minutes BAKE 30 minutes

Nonstick cooking spray

2 teaspoons olive oil

4 bone-in chicken thighs (about 2 pounds total), skin removed

½ cup chopped sweet onion (such as Vidalia or Maui) (1 medium)

½ cup orange juice

2 tablespoons honey

1 tablespoon cornstarch

1 tablespoon Worcestershire sauce

1 tablespoon Dijon-style mustard

1 clove garlic, minced

1 tablespoon sesame oil

9 ounces fresh kale (about 2 bunches), trimmed and coarsely sliced

8 ounces fresh baby portobello mushrooms or button mushrooms, sliced

1 red sweet pepper, coarsely chopped

1 tablespoon rice vinegar

Cracked black pepper (optional)

Orange slices, halved (optional)

PER SERVING: 335 cal., 12 g total fat (2 g sat. fat), 129 mg chol., 264 mg sodium, 27 g carb. (3 g fiber, 17 g sugars), 30 g pro.
Exchanges: 2 vegetable, 1 carb., 4 lean meat, 1 fat.

1 Preheat oven to 375°F. Coat a 2-quart square baking dish with cooking spray. In a very large nonstick skillet heat olive oil over medium-high heat. Add chicken to hot oil; cook about 12 minutes or until browned on all sides, turning to brown evenly. Transfer chicken thighs to the prepared baking dish, arranging in a single layer. Drain drippings from skillet, reserving about 1 teaspoon drippings in skillet.

2 Add onion to hot drippings in skillet; cook and stir for 4 to 5 minutes or until tender, scraping up any browned bits from the bottom of the skillet. In a small bowl whisk together orange juice, honey, cornstarch, Worcestershire sauce, mustard, and garlic; add to skillet. Cook and stir until thickened and bubbly; pour over chicken. Bake about 30 minutes or until chicken is no longer pink (at least 175°F).

3 Meanwhile, use paper towels to wipe out the skillet. Pour sesame oil into skillet; heat over medium-high heat. Add kale, mushrooms, and sweet pepper; cook and stir about 10 minutes or until vegetables are crisp-tender. Add the rice vinegar; toss to combine. To serve, divide kale mixture among four serving plates. Arrange chicken on kale mixture. Whisk the cooking liquid in the bottom of the baking dish until combined; spoon over chicken. If desired, garnish with cracked pepper and orange slices.

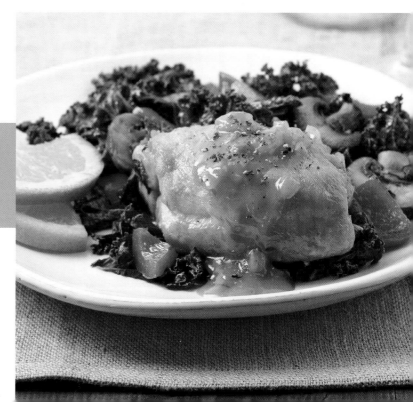

Roasted Chicken with Pistachio Gremolata

For a quick side dish, toss halved and/or whole grape tomatoes in a little of olive oil, snipped fresh herbs, and black pepper.

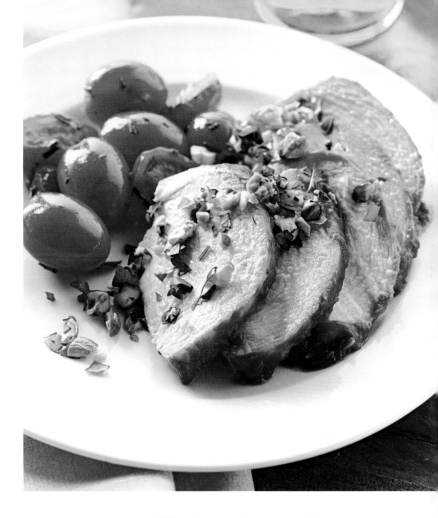

SERVINGS 4 (3 to 4 ounces chicken breast, 2 tablespoons sauce, and 1 tablespoon gremolata each)
CARB. PER SERVING 7 g
PREP 15 minutes **ROAST** 45 minutes

- 2 14- to 16-ounce bone-in chicken breast halves
- 1 teaspoon snipped fresh thyme
- 1/4 teaspoon salt
- 1/8 teaspoon black pepper
- 1/4 cup boiling water
- 2 tablespoons chopped, pitted dates
- 1/4 cup bottled roasted red sweet pepper, drained
- 2 teaspoons balsamic vinegar
- Dash salt
- 1 recipe Pistachio Gremolata

PER SERVING: 191 cal., 5 g total fat (1 g sat. fat), 83 mg chol., 370 mg sodium, 7 g carb. (1 g fiber, 4 g sugars), 28 g pro. Exchanges: 1 vegetable, 3.5 lean meat.

1 Preheat oven to 375°F. Using your fingers, carefully loosen skin from the chicken, making a pocket under the skin while leaving the skin attached. In a small bowl combine thyme, 1/4 teaspoon salt, and the black pepper. Spoon thyme mixture under the skin of the chicken, rubbing it evenly over the meat.

2 Arrange chicken breast halves, skin sides up, in a shallow roasting pan. Roast for 45 to 50 minutes or until chicken is cooked through (at least 170°F).

3 Meanwhile, for sauce, in a small bowl combine boiling water and dates. Cover and let stand for 5 minutes. Transfer date mixture to a blender or small food processor. Add roasted sweet pepper, vinegar, and dash salt. Cover and blend or process until smooth.

4 Remove and discard chicken skin and bones. Brush about half the sauce onto chicken. Slice chicken and place on serving plates. Spoon remaining sauce over chicken. Sprinkle Pistachio Gremolata over chicken to serve.

PISTACHIO GREMOLATA: In a small bowl combine 2 tablespoons snipped fresh parsley, 2 tablespoons chopped shelled pistachio nuts, and 1 small clove garlic, minced.

Chicken Breasts with Lemon-Thyme Cream

Light cream cheese provides silky smoothness and luscious cheesiness to the savory sauce.

SERVINGS 4 (1 chicken breast half and 2 tablespoons sauce each)
CARB. PER SERVING 1 g
PREP 15 minutes **COOK** 35 minutes

Nonstick cooking spray

1 tablespoon olive oil

4 12-ounce bone-in chicken breast halves, skin removed

¼ cup reduced-sodium chicken broth

2 tablespoons fresh lemon juice

½ teaspoon snipped fresh thyme or ⅛ teaspoon dried thyme, crushed

⅛ teaspoon salt

⅛ teaspoon black pepper

2 ounces reduced-fat cream cheese (Neufchâtel), cut up

Snipped fresh thyme (optional)

Lemon wedges or twists (optional)

1 Coat a large nonstick skillet with cooking spray. Add oil and heat over medium-high heat. Add chicken breasts; cook in hot oil about 12 minutes or until golden, turning once halfway through cooking time. Cover and cook about 20 minutes more or until chicken is cooked through (at least 170°F), turning once halfway through cooking time. Remove chicken from skillet; cover with foil and keep warm.

2 In a small bowl stir together chicken broth, lemon juice, ½ teaspoon thyme, the salt, and pepper. Pour broth mixture into the drippings in the hot skillet, scraping up any browned bits from the bottom of the skillet. Add cream cheese and whisk until smooth and heated through. Serve over cooked chicken breasts. If desired, garnish with additional fresh thyme and/or lemon wedges or twists and serve with a green salad.

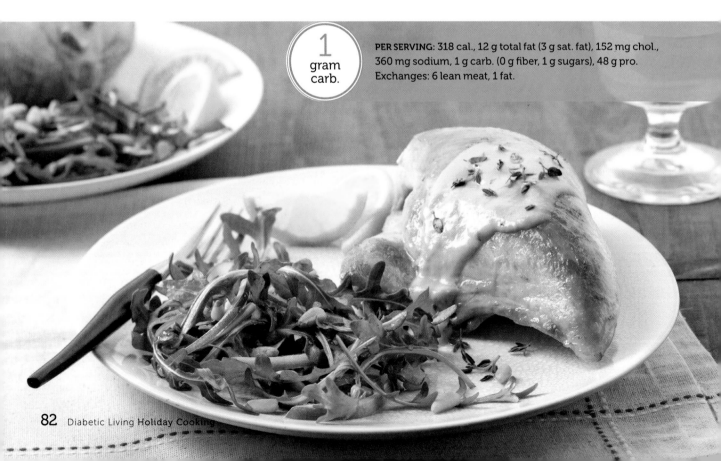

1 gram carb.

PER SERVING: 318 cal., 12 g total fat (3 g sat. fat), 152 mg chol., 360 mg sodium, 1 g carb. (0 g fiber, 1 g sugars), 48 g pro. Exchanges: 6 lean meat, 1 fat.

Grilled Scallops with Pasta and Sherry Cream Sauce

There are lots of pieces, so use long-handled tongs to turn the scallops, Broccolini, and sweet peppers while grilling.

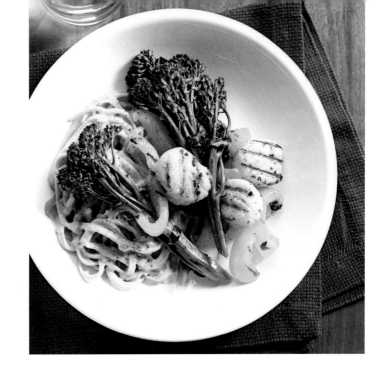

SERVINGS 4 (3 scallops, 1 cup vegetables, and ³/₄ cup pasta mixture each)
CARB. PER SERVING 46 g
PREP 40 minutes   GRILL 10 minutes

12 medium fresh or frozen sea scallops (1¹/₄ pounds total)

1 tablespoon olive oil

¹/₄ teaspoon lemon-pepper seasoning

1 pound Broccolini, trimmed

1 medium yellow or orange sweet pepper, halved

4 ounces dried multigrain or whole grain linguine

1 medium leek, trimmed and thinly sliced

3 cloves garlic, minced

2 teaspoons olive oil

¹/₄ cup dry sherry or apple juice

¹/₃ cup no-salt-added chicken broth

4 teaspoons flour

²/₃ cup fat-free half-and-half

1 tablespoon lemon juice

¹/₈ teaspoon salt

¹/₄ teaspoon crushed red pepper

PER SERVING: 410 cal., 8 g total fat
(1 g sat. fat), 49 mg chol.,
413 mg sodium, 46 g carb. (5 g fiber,
8 g sugars), 34 g pro. Exchanges:
2 vegetable, 2 starch, 3.5 lean meat,
1.5 fat.

1 | Thaw scallops, if frozen. Rinse scallops and pat dry. Brush scallops with 1¹/₂ teaspoons of the olive oil. Sprinkle scallops with the lemon-pepper seasoning. Steam Broccolini for 2 to 3 minutes or until crisp-tender. Drizzle Broccolini and sweet pepper with remaining 1¹/₂ teaspoons oil. Toss to coat. Set scallops, Broccolini, and sweet pepper aside.

2 | Cook linguine according to package directions. Drain, reserving ¹/₂ cup pasta cooking liquid; keep warm.

3 | Meanwhile, in a large skillet cook leek and garlic in the 2 teaspoons olive oil over medium heat for 3 to 5 minutes or just until tender, stirring occasionally. Add sherry. Cook for 2 to 3 minutes or until sherry is nearly evaporated.

4 | In a small bowl whisk together broth and flour until smooth. Add to leek mixture in skillet along with half-and-half, lemon juice, ¹/₄ cup of the pasta cooking liquid, the salt, and crushed red pepper. Cook and stir over medium heat until thickened and bubbly. Cook and stir for 1 minute more. Add drained linguine and toss to coat. Cover and keep warm. Stir in additional reserved pasta cooking liquid as needed to reach desired sauce consistency.

5 | For a charcoal or gas grill, place Broccolini, pepper halves, and scallops on the greased grill rack directly over medium heat. Cover; grill pepper halves for 8 to 10 minutes or until crisp-tender, turning once. Grill scallops for 5 to 8 minutes or until opaque, turning once halfway through grilling. Grill Broccolini for 3 to 5 minutes or until crisp-tender, turning once. Cut pepper into bite-size strips.

6 | Divide pasta mixture among four serving plates. Top with grilled vegetables and scallops.

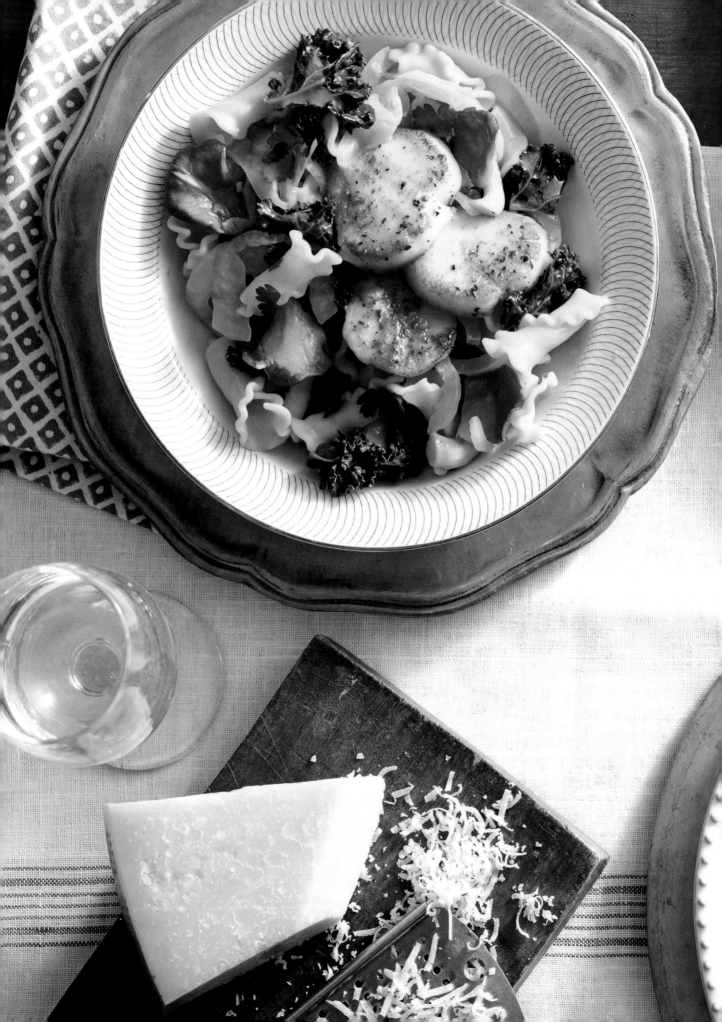

Scallop, Mushroom, and Fennel Campanelle

Oyster mushrooms get their name because they look, smell, and taste like oysters. If they are not available, use other fresh mushrooms.

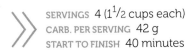

SERVINGS 4 (1½ cups each)
CARB. PER SERVING 42 g
START TO FINISH 40 minutes

8 ounces fresh or frozen sea scallops
6 ounces dried campanelle pasta
¼ teaspoon salt
¼ teaspoon black pepper
3 teaspoons olive oil
2 cups fresh oyster mushrooms, cut into 2-inch pieces
2 cloves garlic, minced
2 cups chopped kale
1½ cups thinly sliced fennel
¼ cup dry white wine
¼ cup light butter with canola oil
2 tablespoons snipped fresh parsley
2 tablespoons lemon juice
⅛ teaspoon salt

1 | Thaw scallops, if frozen. Rinse scallops; pat dry with paper towels. Cut scallops horizontally in half. In a large saucepan cook pasta according to package directions. Drain; set aside.

2 | Sprinkle scallops with the ¼ teaspoon salt and the pepper. In a large nonstick skillet heat 1 teaspoon of the olive oil over medium heat. Add scallops; cook for 2 to 3 minutes or until scallops are opaque, turning once. Remove from skillet; keep warm. Add another 1 teaspoon of the oil, the mushrooms, and garlic. Cook about 4 minutes or until mushrooms are tender. Remove from skillet; keep warm. Add the remaining 1 teaspoon oil, the kale, and fennel. Cook about 7 minutes more or just until kale and fennel are tender.

3 | Remove skillet from heat and add wine. Return to heat. Add butter, parsley, lemon juice, and the ⅛ teaspoon salt; stir to combine. Add the cooked pasta and the mushroom mixture to the butter mixture; toss to combine. Heat through. To serve, divide pasta-mushroom mixture among four serving bowls; place scallops on top of pasta-mushroom mixture.

PER SERVING: 331 cal., 10 g total fat (3 g sat. fat), 19 mg chol., 567 mg sodium, 42 g carb. (4 g fiber, 3 g sugars), 16 g pro. Exchanges: 2 vegetable, 2 starch, 1.5 lean meat, 1.5 fat.

10 grams fat

Coconut-Curry Salmon with Lentils

If you prefer your salmon slightly pink in the center, start checking it for doneness a couple minutes early.

SERVINGS 4 (1 salmon fillet and $^2/_3$ cup lentil mixture each)
CARB. PER SERVING 21 g
PREP 20 minutes   COOK 12 minutes
BAKE 10 minutes

- 4 4-ounce fresh or frozen skinless salmon fillets
- $^1/_2$ teaspoon curry powder
- $^1/_4$ teaspoon salt
- $^1/_4$ teaspoon black pepper
- $^1/_4$ cup unsweetened flaked or shredded coconut
- 2 tablespoons panko bread crumbs
- Olive oil nonstick cooking spray
- $^3/_4$ cup reduced-sodium chicken broth or vegetable broth
- $^1/_4$ cup unsweetened light coconut milk
- 2 cups cauliflower florets
- $^1/_2$ cup dry red lentils
- 3 cloves garlic, minced
- 2 tablespoons snipped fresh mint

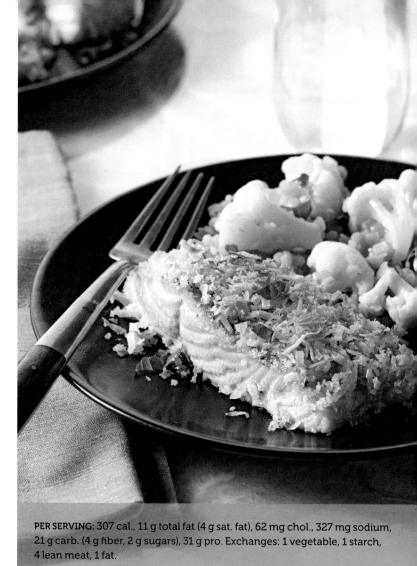

PER SERVING: 307 cal., 11 g total fat (4 g sat. fat), 62 mg chol., 327 mg sodium, 21 g carb. (4 g fiber, 2 g sugars), 31 g pro. Exchanges: 1 vegetable, 1 starch, 4 lean meat, 1 fat.

1 Thaw salmon, if frozen. Preheat oven to 425°F. Rinse fish; pat dry with paper towels. Place salmon on a parchment paper-lined baking sheet.

2 In a small bowl combine curry powder, salt, and pepper. Sprinkle evenly on salmon. In the same small bowl combine the flaked coconut and bread crumbs. Spoon evenly over top of salmon. Lightly coat coconut topping with cooking spray.

3 Bake salmon for 10 to 15 minutes or until fish flakes easily when tested with a fork.

4 Meanwhile, in a medium saucepan bring broth and coconut milk to boiling. Add cauliflower, lentils, and garlic. Reduce heat; cover and simmer about 12 minutes or until lentils and cauliflower are tender. Divide lentils and salmon among four shallow bowls. To serve, sprinkle with mint.

Smoky-Hot Raspberry Shrimp

Use a knife to cut iceberg or romaine lettuce into shreds. For a quicker option, purchase a bag of shredded lettuce.

SERVINGS 4 (6 to 8 cooked shrimp, 1 cup lettuce, 1/4 cup jicama, and 1 tablespoon sauce each)
CARB. PER SERVING 29 g
START TO FINISH 30 minutes

- 12 ounces fresh or frozen medium shrimp
- 1 8-ounce can pineapple chunks (juice pack)
- 2 teaspoons chili powder
- 1 teaspoon ground cumin
- 1/2 teaspoon coarsely ground black pepper
- 1/3 cup raspberry spreadable fruit
- 1 1/2 teaspoons Worcestershire sauce
- 1 teaspoon chopped canned chipotle chile peppers in adobo sauce (see tip, *page 71*)

Nonstick cooking spray

- 4 cups shredded lettuce
- 1/2 of a small jicama, peeled and cut into matchstick-size strips (1 cup)
- 1 tablespoon shredded coconut, toasted

1 Thaw shrimp, if frozen. Peel and devein shrimp, leaving tails intact if desired. Rinse shrimp; pat dry with paper towels. Drain pineapple, reserving 3 tablespoons of the juice; set aside. In a small bowl combine chili powder, cumin, and black pepper. Sprinkle spice mixture evenly over shrimp; rub in with your fingers.

2 For sauce, in a small microwave-safe bowl combine raspberry spreadable fruit, 2 tablespoons of the reserved pineapple juice, the Worcestershire sauce, and chile peppers. Microwave on 100 percent power (high) about 1 minute or until spreadable fruit is melted. Stir until smooth. Set aside 1/4 cup of the sauce for drizzling.

3 Lightly coat a grill pan with cooking spray; heat over medium-high heat. Add the shrimp; cook about 5 minutes or until nearly opaque, turning occasionally. Brush the remaining sauce over both sides of the shrimp and add pineapple to pan; cook shrimp and pineapple for 1 minute more. Discard any remaining sauce used as a brush-on.

4 On a serving platter or plates arrange lettuce and jicama. Top with shrimp and pineapple. Stir the remaining 1 tablespoon pineapple juice into the reserved sauce; drizzle over all on platter. Sprinkle with coconut.

PER SERVING: 180 cal., 2 g total fat (1 g sat. fat), 107 mg chol., 536 mg sodium, 29 g carb. (4 g fiber, 21 g sugars), 13 g pro. Exchanges: 1 vegetable, 1.5 fruit, 2 lean meat.

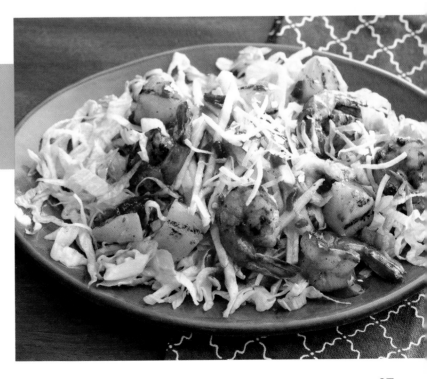

Quinoa Crab Cakes with Asian Slaw

Look for white miso paste in the Asian section of the supermarket or take a trip to an Asian food market.

SERVINGS 2 (2 crab cakes and about $^1/_2$ cup slaw each)
CARB. PER SERVING 15 g
PREP 25 minutes COOK 8 minutes

- 2 teaspoons white miso paste
- 2 teaspoons rice vinegar
- 1 teaspoon honey
- $^1/_2$ cup purchased shredded carrot
- $^1/_3$ cup coarsely shredded radishes
- $^1/_3$ cup fresh sugar snap peas, trimmed and thinly sliced lengthwise
- 1 green onion, thinly sliced
- 2 tablespoons refrigerated or frozen egg product, thawed, or 1 egg white, lightly beaten
- $^1/_4$ cup cooked quinoa
- 2 tablespoons plain low-fat or fat-free yogurt
- $^1/_2$ teaspoon grated fresh ginger
- $^1/_4$ teaspoon ground coriander
- $^1/_8$ teaspoon ground cumin
- $^1/_8$ teaspoon cayenne pepper
- $^1/_8$ teaspoon ground turmeric
- 1 cup cooked lump crabmeat, cartilage removed, or one 6-ounce can crabmeat, drained, flaked, and cartilage removed

Nonstick cooking spray

- 2 teaspoons canola oil

1 For slaw, in a medium bowl whisk together miso, vinegar, and honey. Add carrot, radishes, peas, and green onion. Toss to coat. Let stand at room temperature while preparing crab cakes.

2 For crab cakes, in a medium bowl combine egg, quinoa, yogurt, ginger, coriander, cumin, cayenne pepper, and turmeric. Add crabmeat; mix well. Using moistened hands, shape crab mixture into four $^1/_2$-inch-thick patties.

3 Coat a large nonstick skillet with cooking spray and add oil. Heat over medium heat. Add crab cakes. Cook for 8 minutes or until golden brown and heated through, carefully turning once with a thin-bladed metal spatula. Serve crab cakes with the slaw.

PER SERVING: 189 cal., 6 g total fat (1 g sat. fat), 104 mg chol., 578 mg sodium, 15 g carb. (2 g fiber, 7 g sugars), 19 g pro. Exchanges: 1 vegetable, 0.5 starch, 2 lean meat, 1 fat.

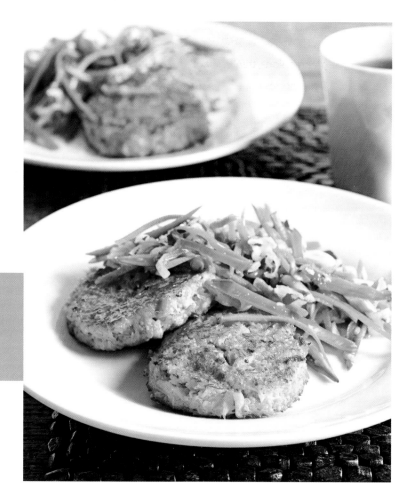

Cheesy Butternut Squash and Cavatappi Bake

The peel on the butternut squash can be hard to remove. Use a sharp vegetable peeler or a sharp paring knife to remove one strip at a time.

SERVINGS 8 (1 cup each)
CARB. PER SERVING 32 g
PREP 30 minutes MICROWAVE 8 minutes
BAKE 20 minutes

Nonstick cooking spray

3 cups cubed, peeled butternut squash (at least 1¾ pounds squash)

2 tablespoons water

8 ounces dried cavatappi or elbow macaroni (about 3 cups)

1 tablespoon butter

8 ounces fresh cremini or button mushrooms, sliced (3 cups)

3 green onions, thinly sliced

2 tablespoons flour

1 cup fat-free milk

¼ teaspoon salt

¼ teaspoon black pepper

1½ cups shredded part-skim mozzarella cheese (6 ounces)

2 slices lower-sodium, less-fat bacon, cooked and crumbled

Thinly sliced green onions (optional)

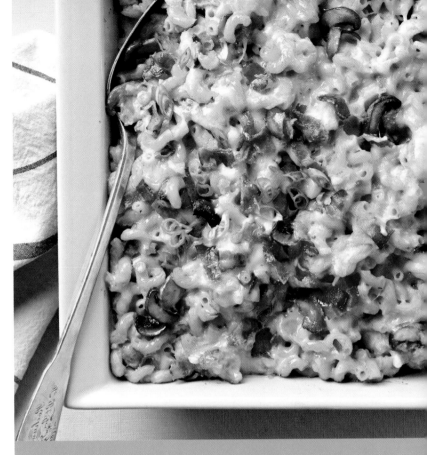

PER SERVING: 227 cal., 6 g total fat (3 g sat. fat), 19 mg chol., 254 mg sodium, 32 g carb. (2 g fiber, 4 g sugars), 12 g pro. Exchanges: 2 starch, 1 lean meat, 0.5 fat.

1 Preheat oven to 375°F. Lightly coat a 2-quart rectangular baking dish with cooking spray; set aside.

2 In a medium microwave-safe bowl combine squash and the water; cover with vented plastic wrap. Microwave on 100 percent power (high) for 4 minutes; stir. Microwave, covered, about 4 minutes more or until squash is tender. Carefully remove plastic wrap. Mash squash; set aside.

3 Meanwhile, cook pasta according to package directions; drain. In a medium saucepan heat butter over medium heat. Add mushrooms and green onions. Cook about 5 minutes or until tender. Sprinkle flour over mushroom mixture. Cook and stir for 1 minute. Add milk, salt, and pepper. Cook and stir over medium heat until thickened and bubbly. Remove from heat; stir in squash. Add pasta; gently fold to combine.

4 Transfer half of the pasta mixture to the prepared baking dish. Sprinkle with half of the cheese. Add remaining pasta mixture and cheese. Top with bacon.

5 Bake, uncovered, for 20 to 25 minutes or until heated through and cheese is melted. If desired, top with additional green onions.

Spinach Alfredo Lasagna

To drain the spinach, place it in a fine-mesh sieve and use the back of a spoon to press on the spinach to squeeze out excess water.

SERVINGS 8 (1 piece [$^1/_8$ of the lasagna] each)
CARB. PER SERVING 24 g
PREP 25 minutes   BAKE 1 hour 15 minutes   STAND 20 minutes

Nonstick cooking spray

1 egg, lightly beaten

1 15-ounce carton part-skim ricotta cheese

1 10-ounce package frozen chopped spinach, thawed and well drained

4 cloves garlic, minced

$^1/_4$ teaspoon freshly ground black pepper

1 15-ounce jar light Alfredo sauce

$^1/_2$ cup fat-free milk

6 whole grain lasagna noodles

2 cups shredded carrots (4 medium)

2 cups sliced fresh mushrooms

$^1/_2$ cup shredded part-skim mozzarella cheese (2 ounces)

$^1/_4$ cup finely shredded Parmesan cheese (1 ounce)

1 Preheat oven to 350°F. Lightly coat a 2-quart rectangular baking dish with cooking spray.

2 In a medium bowl stir together egg, ricotta cheese, spinach, garlic, and pepper. In a separate bowl combine Alfredo sauce and milk.

3 Spread about $^1/_2$ cup of the Alfredo sauce mixture in the bottom of the prepared baking dish. Arrange three of the uncooked noodles in a layer over the sauce. Spread half of the spinach mixture over the noodles; top with half of the carrots and half of the mushrooms. Arrange the remaining three uncooked noodles over the vegetables. Top noodles with the remaining spinach mixture. Top with the remaining carrots and the remaining mushrooms. Cover with the remaining Alfredo mixture. Sprinkle with the mozzarella cheese and Parmesan cheese.

4 Lightly coat a sheet of foil with cooking spray. Cover dish with foil, coated side down.

5 Bake for 60 to 70 minutes. Uncover. Bake for 15 to 20 minutes more or until top is lightly browned. Let stand for 20 minutes. Cut into eight pieces.

16 grams pro.

PER SERVING: 262 cal., 12 g total fat (7 g sat. fat), 69 mg chol., 527 mg sodium, 24 g carb. (4 g fiber, 4 g sugars), 16 g pro. Exchanges: 2 vegetable, 1 starch, 1.5 lean meat, 1.5 fat.

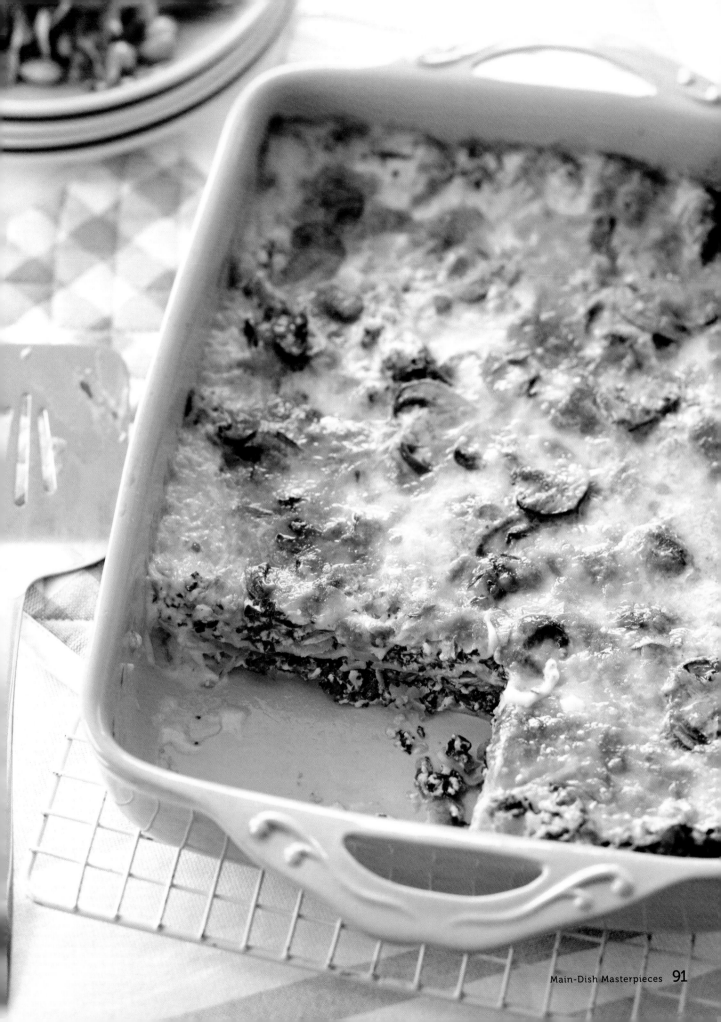

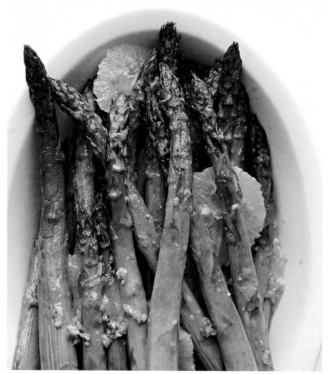
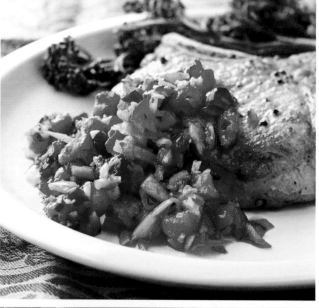
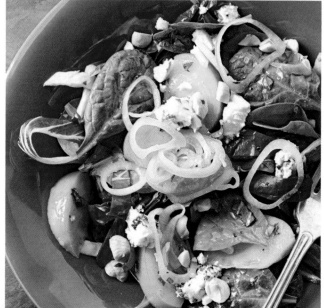

seasonal
sides and salads

Holiday meal planning often begins around a golden bird, juicy

roast, or succulent shellfish. But side dishes bring the party to

the palate. Fresh produce packs a powerful punch with both

flavor and nutrition, so try one of these new recipes—each will

delight your taste buds and add health benefits.

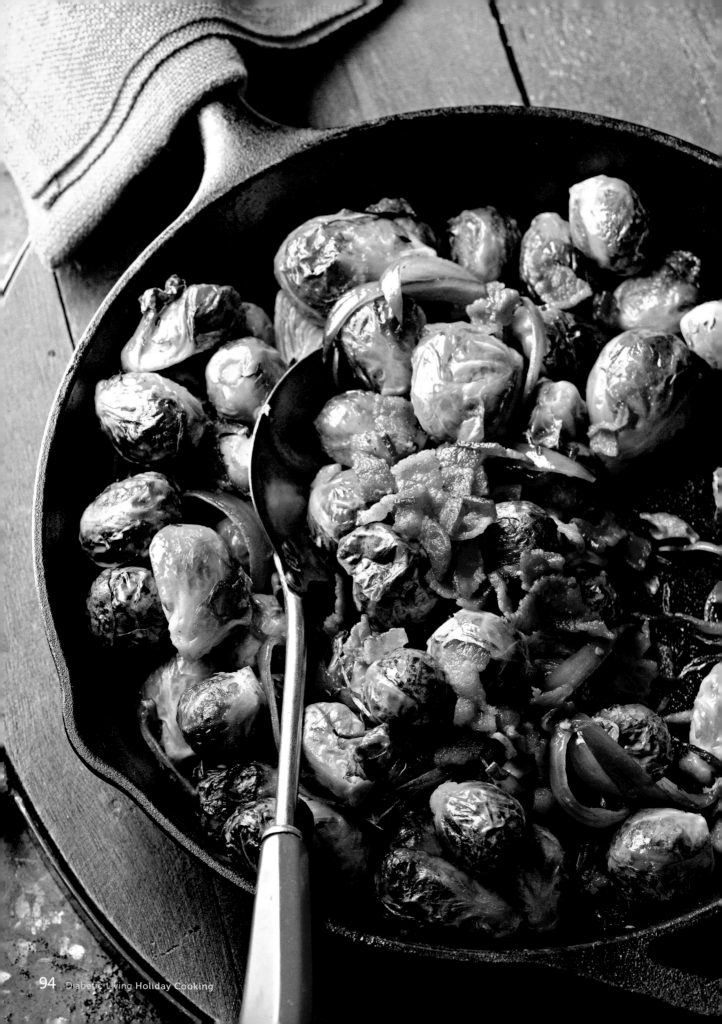

Bacon-Roasted Brussels Sprouts

Try lower-sodium, less-fat bacon when a recipe calls for bacon. This pork product has more than 30 percent less sodium and fat than traditional bacon and tastes great, too!

SERVINGS 8 ($^2/_3$ cup each)
CARB. PER SERVING 11 g
PREP 15 minutes **ROAST** 20 minutes

2 slices bacon, cut crosswise into thin strips

$^1/_8$ teaspoon crushed red pepper

2 pounds Brussels sprouts, trimmed

$^1/_2$ cup thin wedges red onion

2 teaspoons fresh thyme leaves

$^1/_4$ teaspoon salt

1 Preheat oven to 400°F. In a very large cast-iron or other heavy oven-going skillet cook and stir bacon over medium heat until bacon is browned and crisp. Using a slotted spoon, remove bacon to paper towels to drain. Add crushed red pepper to drippings in skillet; cook and stir for 1 minute or until fragrant.

2 If Brussels sprouts are large, halve lengthwise. Add sprouts, onion, thyme, and salt to skillet. Stir to coat with drippings. Transfer skillet to oven and roast mixture, uncovered, for 20 to 25 minutes or until sprouts are just tender and browned, stirring once.

3 Transfer sprouts and onion to a serving dish and sprinkle with reserved bacon.

PER SERVING: 93 cal., 4 g total fat (1 g sat. fat), 6 mg chol., 164 mg sodium, 11 g carb. (5 g fiber, 3 g sugars), 5 g pro. Exchanges: 2 vegetable, 1 fat.

11 grams carb.

QUICK TIP
To trim Brussels sprouts, cut off the stems just at the spot where the leaves start to grow. Remove dark green outer leaves until the tender, light green leaves are uniformly exposed.

Soy- and Chile-Glazed Brussels Sprouts with Shiitake Mushrooms

If the Brussels sprouts are difficult to stir, use a spatula to flip them so they cook evenly.

SERVINGS 5 (²/₃ cup each)
CARB. PER SERVING 14 g
START TO FINISH 40 minutes

- 1 pound Brussels sprouts, trimmed (see tip, *page 95*)
- 4 green onions
- 1 teaspoon finely shredded orange peel
- 2 tablespoons orange juice
- 1 tablespoon reduced-sodium soy sauce
- 1½ teaspoons honey
- ½ of a fresh red serrano chile pepper, seeded and finely chopped, (see tip, *page 71*) or ¼ teaspoon crushed red pepper
- 1 to 2 cloves garlic, minced
- 1½ tablespoons vegetable oil
- 4 ounces fresh shiitake mushrooms, stemmed and thinly sliced

1 Cut trimmed sprouts lengthwise into quarters. Finely chop one of the green onions; cut the remaining three green onions diagonally into 1-inch pieces. In a small bowl stir together orange peel, orange juice, soy sauce, honey, serrano pepper, and garlic; set aside.

2 Working in a well-ventilated area, in a large skillet heat oil over medium-high heat. Add Brussels sprouts, green onions, and mushrooms. Cook and stir for 8 to 10 minutes or until sprouts are blackened in places and are nearly tender.

3 Pour orange juice mixture over sprout mixture; toss to coat. Cook and stir for 3 to 4 minutes more or until sprouts are tender.

PER SERVING: 100 cal., 5 g total fat (1 g sat. fat), 0 mg chol., 137 mg sodium, 14 g carb. (4 g fiber, 6 g sugars), 4 g pro. Exchanges: 2 vegetable, 1 fat.

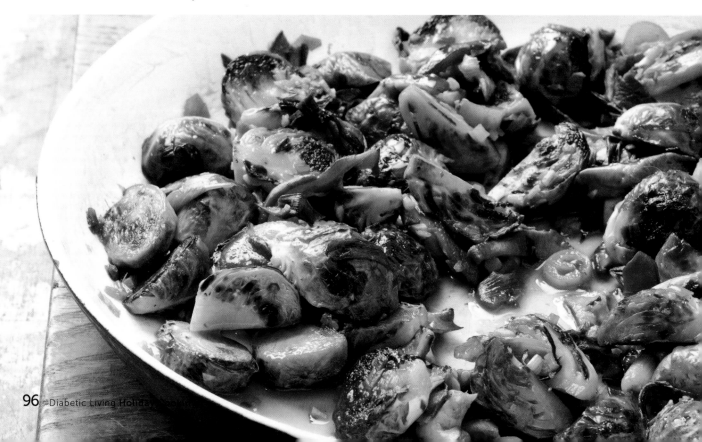

Roasted Asparagus-Orange Salad

Dressed with orange slices and citrus vinaigrette, warm roasted asparagus evolves from a simple side dish to a holiday meal star.

SERVINGS 8 (4 ounces asparagus and 2 teaspoons dressing each)
CARB. PER SERVING 6 g
PREP 10 minutes
ROAST 15 minutes

2 pounds green, white, and/or purple asparagus spears, trimmed

1 tablespoon olive oil

¼ teaspoon salt

2 oranges

1 clove garlic, minced

1 teaspoon Dijon-style mustard

½ teaspoon fennel seeds, crushed

2 tablespoons olive oil

1 tablespoon cider vinegar

QUICK TIP
Starting at the base of each spear and working toward the tip, bend the spear a few times until you find a place where it breaks easily. Snap off the woody base at that point.

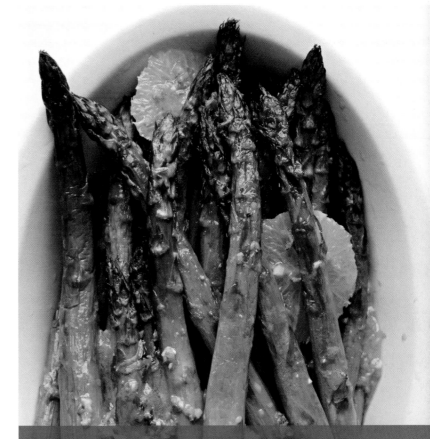

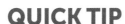

PER SERVING: 74 cal., 5 g total fat (1 g sat. fat), 0 mg chol., 89 mg sodium, 6 g carb. (2 g fiber, 4 g sugars), 2 g pro. Exchanges: 0.5 vegetable, 1 fat.

1 Preheat oven to 400°F. Place asparagus in a 15×10×1-inch baking pan. Drizzle with the 1 tablespoon oil and sprinkle with the salt; toss to coat. Roast, uncovered, for 15 to 20 minutes until asparagus is crisp-tender, tossing once. Transfer to a serving platter.

2 Meanwhile, for dressing, shred enough peel from one orange to equal 1 teaspoon; set aside. Squeeze juice from half of an orange. Peel, then slice the remaining half and whole orange into rounds. In a jar with a tight-fitting lid combine the shredded orange peel, orange juice, garlic, mustard, fennel seeds, 2 tablespoons oil, and the vinegar. Cover with lid and shake to combine.

3 Drizzle a little of the dressing on the asparagus; toss to coat. Carefully toss in orange slices. Pass any remaining dressing.

Acorn Squash with Bacon-Chive Crumbs

Grab your slow cooker and let it give you a hand at cooking this holiday. The squash cooks for several hours, giving you time to work on other components of the meal.

SERVINGS 8 ($^1/_4$ of a squash and 1$^1/_2$ tablespoons panko mixture each)
CARB. PER SERVING 17 g or 15 g
PREP 25 minutes   SLOW COOK 4 to 5 hours (low) or 2 to 3 hours (high)

- 2 medium acorn squash (2$^1/_2$ to 3 pounds total)
- 4 cloves garlic
- 3 sprigs fresh thyme
- $^3/_4$ cup apple cider
- $^1/_2$ cup reduced-sodium chicken broth or vegetable broth
- 2 tablespoons packed brown sugar*
- 3 slices bacon
- $^1/_3$ cup panko bread crumbs
- 3 tablespoons snipped fresh chives

1 Cut $^1/_2$ inch off the top and bottom of each squash; cut each squash in half lengthwise. Remove and discard seeds. Cut each squash half crosswise into $^1/_2$-inch-thick slices.

2 Layer squash slices in a 4- to 5-quart slow cooker. Add garlic and thyme. In a 2-cup glass measure stir together cider, broth, and brown sugar. Pour over squash in cooker.

3 Cover and cook on low-heat setting for 4 to 5 hours or on high-heat setting for 2 to 3 hours. Rearrange slices halfway through cooking.

4 Just before serving, in a large skillet cook bacon over medium heat for 5 to 7 minutes or until crisp. Transfer bacon to paper towels to drain; discard drippings. (Do not wipe skillet clean.) Finely crumble bacon. Heat skillet over medium-high heat. Add panko; cook and stir for 1 to 2 minutes or until golden. Transfer toasted panko to a bowl; cool. Stir bacon and chives into panko.

5 To serve, transfer squash to a serving platter. Sprinkle with panko mixture.

*SUGAR SUBSTITUTE: Choose Splenda Brown Sugar Blend for Baking. Follow package directions to use product amount equivalent to 2 tablespoons brown sugar.

MAKE-AHEAD DIRECTIONS: Prepare squash as directed in Step 1. Place squash slices in a resealable plastic bag; chill for up to 24 hours.

PER SERVING: 98 cal., 2 g total fat (1 g sat. fat), 4 mg chol., 99 mg sodium, 17 g carb. (2 g fiber, 4 g sugars), 3 g pro. Exchanges: 1 starch, 0.5 fat.

PER SERVING WITH SUBSTITUTE: Same as above, except 93 cal., 15 g carb. (2 g sugars), 98 mg sodium.

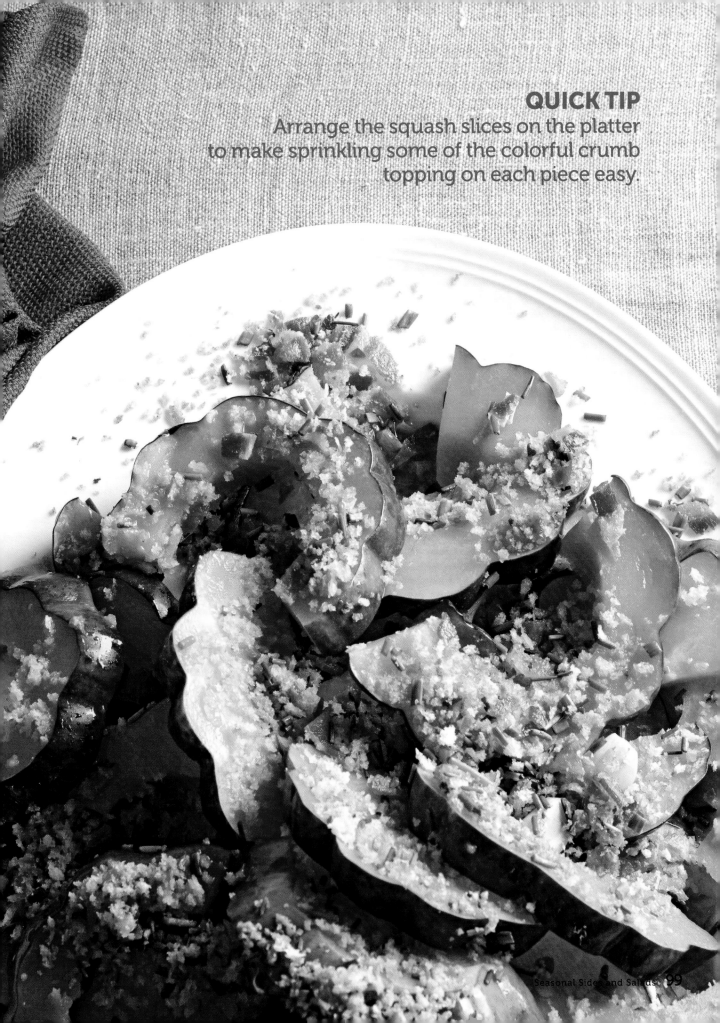

QUICK TIP
Arrange the squash slices on the platter
to make sprinkling some of the colorful crumb
topping on each piece easy.

Broccoli with Peas and Seared Lemons

Broccolini makes a pretty substitute for broccoli—the florets are frilly and the stems are long and slender.

SERVINGS 12 (¹/₂ cup each)
CARB. PER SERVING 6 g
START TO FINISH 30 minutes

- 2 pounds broccoli or Broccolini, trimmed
- 8 ounces Swiss chard, trimmed and cut into 2- to 3-inch lengths
- 1 cup frozen peas
- 2 tablespoons butter
- 1 lemon, thinly sliced
- ¹/₄ cup chicken broth
- ¹/₄ teaspoon crushed red pepper
- ¹/₄ cup snipped fresh chives
- ¹/₂ teaspoon coarse salt

QUICK TIP
To ensure a nice sear, do not move the lemon slices around too much during cooking.

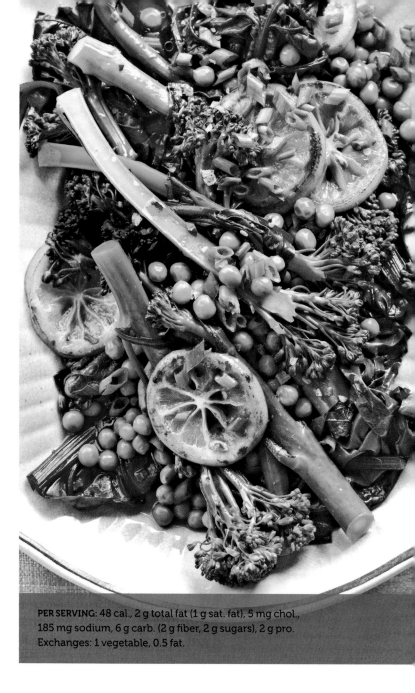

PER SERVING: 48 cal., 2 g total fat (1 g sat. fat), 5 mg chol., 185 mg sodium, 6 g carb. (2 g fiber, 2 g sugars), 2 g pro.
Exchanges: 1 vegetable, 0.5 fat.

1 Bring a large pot of salted water to boiling. Add broccoli; cook for 2 minutes. Add Swiss chard and peas. Cover and simmer about 4 minutes or until bright green; drain.

2 Meanwhile, melt butter in a large skillet over medium to medium-high heat. Add lemon slices; cook about 3 minutes per side or until lemons are soft and browned and butter is browned.

3 Return drained broccoli, chard, and peas to the pot. Add the broth and crushed red pepper; toss gently to coat. Transfer the broccoli mixture to a serving platter. Top with the lemon slices, chives, and salt.

Creamy Smashed Turnips

Cut the cream cheese into small cubes before adding it to the mashed turnips. This will help distribute the cheese and make mashing easier.

SERVINGS 4 (²/₃ cup each)
CARB. PER SERVING 10 g
PREP 20 minutes **COOK** 25 minutes

1½ pounds turnips (2 large), peeled and cut into ½-inch cubes (5 cups)

2 ounces reduced-fat cream cheese (Neufchâtel), softened

¼ teaspoon garlic powder

¼ teaspoon black pepper

⅛ teaspoon kosher salt

Fresh chives

1 Bring a large saucepan or pot of water to boiling; add cubed turnips. Return to boiling; reduce heat. Simmer, covered, about 25 minutes or until turnips are very tender. Drain well; return turnips to the hot saucepan.

2 Using a potato masher, mash turnips until nearly smooth. Add cream cheese; mash until combined.

3 Stir in garlic powder, pepper, and salt. Garnish with chives. Serve warm.

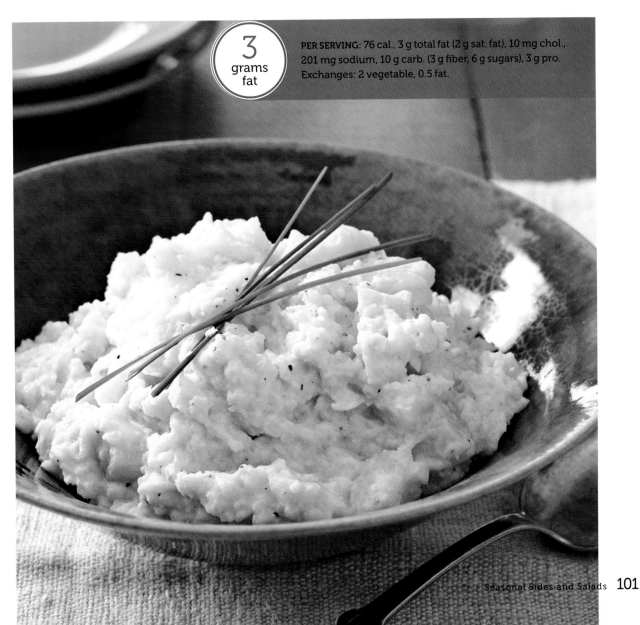

3 grams fat

PER SERVING: 76 cal., 3 g total fat (2 g sat. fat), 10 mg chol., 201 mg sodium, 10 g carb. (3 g fiber, 6 g sugars), 3 g pro. Exchanges: 2 vegetable, 0.5 fat.

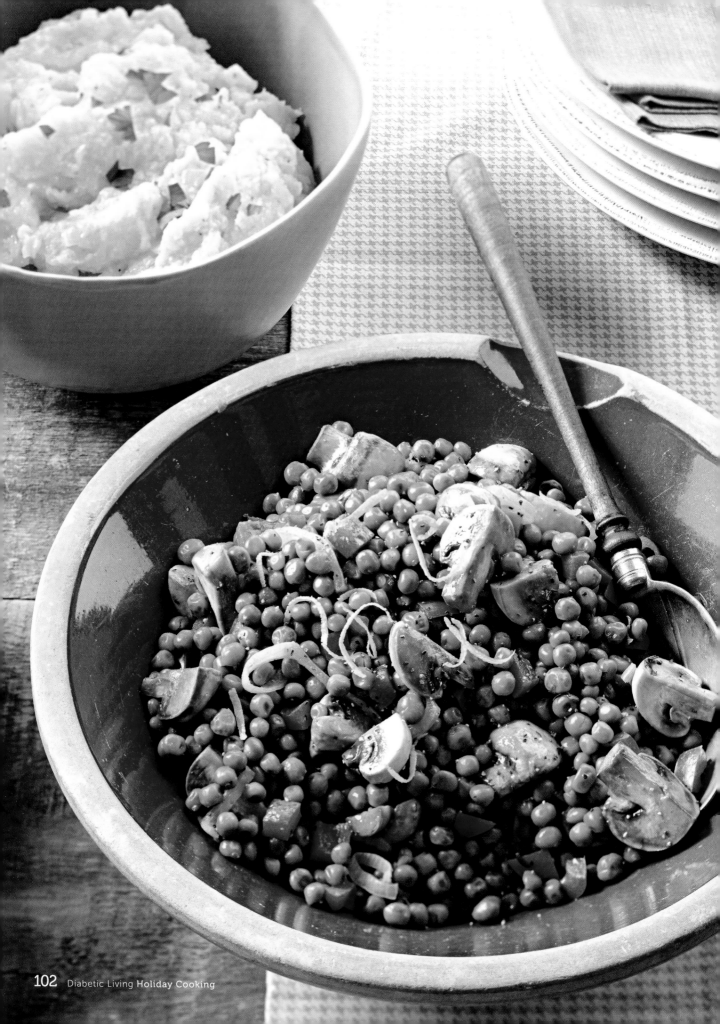

Parsley Mashed Potatoes

Adding cauliflower to family-favorite mashed potatoes is a great way to give them a boost—cauliflower is loaded with disease-fighting antioxidants.

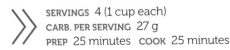

SERVINGS 4 (1 cup each)
CARB. PER SERVING 27 g
PREP 25 minutes **COOK** 25 minutes

- 12 ounces Yukon gold potatoes (about 3), peeled and cubed
- 6 cups cauliflower florets
- 1/2 cup chopped onion (1 medium)
- 1 tablespoon butter
- 1/4 teaspoon kosher salt
- 1/4 teaspoon black pepper
- 2 tablespoons snipped fresh parsley

1 In a covered 4- to 5-quart Dutch oven cook potatoes, cauliflower, and onion in boiling water about 25 minutes or until very tender. Drain mixture. Transfer to a large bowl.

2 Beat with an electric mixer on medium speed until nearly smooth. Beat in butter, salt, and pepper. Stir in parsley just before serving.

PER SERVING: 145 cal., 3 g total fat (2 g sat. fat), 8 mg chol., 199 mg sodium, 27 g carb. (5 g fiber, 4 g sugars), 5 g pro. Exchanges: 2 vegetable, 1 starch, 0.5 fat.

Peas with Mushrooms, Shallots, and Red Sweet Pepper

Experiment with the flavor of this dish by changing the herb—try fresh basil, thyme, and oregano as other options.

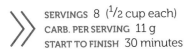

SERVINGS 8 (1/2 cup each)
CARB. PER SERVING 11 g
START TO FINISH 30 minutes

- 2 tablespoons butter
- 8 ounces whole fresh button or cremini mushrooms, quartered
- 3/4 cup chopped red sweet pepper (1 medium)
- 1/4 cup coarsely chopped shallots (2 medium) or sweet onion
- 1 16-ounce package frozen petite peas, thawed
- 1/4 teaspoon black pepper
- 1/8 teaspoon salt
- 1 tablespoon snipped fresh tarragon or mint
- 2 teaspoons finely shredded lemon peel

1 In a large skillet melt butter over medium heat. Add mushrooms, sweet pepper, and shallots; cook about 5 minutes or until tender but not browned, stirring occasionally. Stir in the peas, pepper, and salt. Cook about 5 minutes or until peas are tender, stirring occasionally. Stir in tarragon. Transfer to a serving bowl. Sprinkle with lemon peel.

PER SERVING: 86 cal., 3 g total fat (2 g sat. fat), 8 mg chol., 195 mg sodium, 11 g carb. (3 g fiber, 4 g sugars), 4 g pro. Exchanges: 0.5 vegetable, 0.5 starch, 0.5 fat.

Honey 'n' Spice Sweet Potatoes with Toasted Coconut

To toast coconut, spread flakes in a shallow baking pan. Bake at 350°F for 5 to 10 minutes, shaking pan once or twice. Watch closely to prevent burning.

SERVINGS 6 (½ cup each)
CARB. PER SERVING 24 g
PREP 15 minutes   COOK 12 minutes

- 1½   pounds sweet potatoes, peeled and cut into 1-inch pieces
- ½   cup unsweetened light coconut milk
- 1   tablespoon coconut oil or canola oil*
- 2   tablespoons honey
- ½   teaspoon pumpkin pie spice
- ⅓   cup unsweetened shredded or flaked coconut, toasted

1 Place sweet potatoes in a steamer basket. Place basket in a very large skillet over 1 inch of boiling water. Steam the sweet potatoes, covered, for 8 to 10 minutes or until just tender. Remove steamer basket with sweet potatoes. Pour water out of skillet; carefully wipe skillet dry.

2 In the skillet combine coconut milk, oil, honey, and pumpkin pie spice. Bring to boiling; reduce heat. Add sweet potato pieces. Simmer, uncovered, for 4 to 6 minutes or until potatoes are well coated and most of the liquid is absorbed, stirring often.

3 To serve, transfer sweet potatoes to a serving dish. Sprinkle with toasted coconut.

*TEST KITCHEN TIP: If you use the tablespoon measure for the oil before using it to measure the honey, the oil-coated spoon will help the honey come out of the measuring spoon easier.

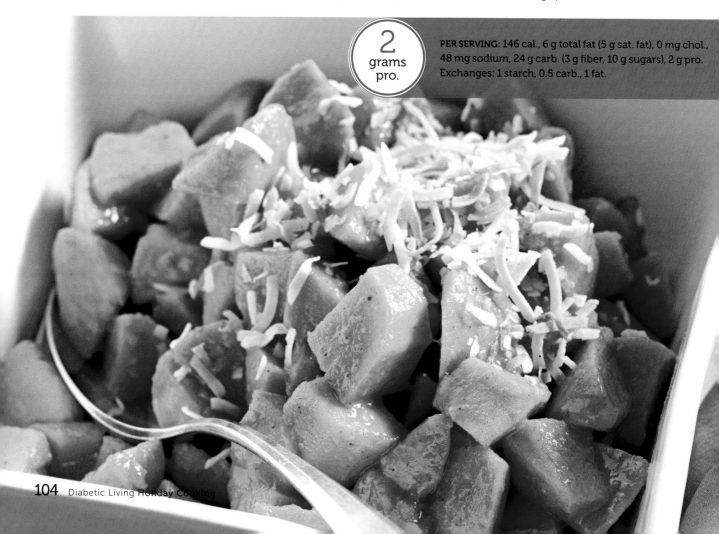

2 grams pro.

PER SERVING: 146 cal., 6 g total fat (5 g sat. fat), 0 mg chol., 48 mg sodium, 24 g carb. (3 g fiber, 10 g sugars), 2 g pro. Exchanges: 1 starch, 0.5 carb., 1 fat.

Lemon-Garlic Mashed Potatoes

Not your typical mashed potatoes—leave these skin-on potatoes on the chunky side instead of mashing until smooth and creamy.

SERVINGS 16 (¹/₂ cup each)
CARB. PER SERVING 14 g
PREP 20 minutes **COOK** 20 minutes

- 3 pounds Yukon gold potatoes, scrubbed and cut into chunks
- 4 cloves garlic, halved
- 3 tablespoons olive oil
- 2 tablespoons butter
- ¹/₂ teaspoon salt
- ¹/₄ teaspoon freshly ground black pepper
- 2 tablespoons capers, drained and chopped
- ¹/₃ cup chopped fresh Italian (flat-leaf) parsley
- 2 teaspoons finely shredded lemon peel
- 1 lemon half

QUICK TIP
Olive oil stars in the overall flavor of this dish, so choose one that pleases your palate.

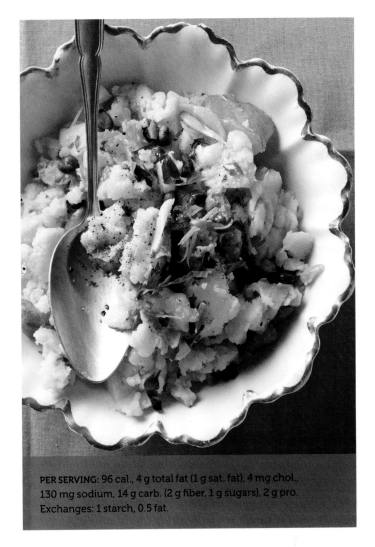

PER SERVING: 96 cal., 4 g total fat (1 g sat. fat), 4 mg chol., 130 mg sodium, 14 g carb. (2 g fiber, 1 g sugars), 2 g pro. Exchanges: 1 starch, 0.5 fat.

1 In a large saucepan cook potatoes and garlic in lightly salted boiling water, covered, for 20 to 25 minutes or until tender.

2 Drain potatoes, reserving 1 cup water. Using a potato masher, mash potatoes to desired consistency. Add 2 tablespoons of the olive oil, the butter, salt, pepper, and enough of the reserved liquid to reach desired consistency. Stir to combine. Transfer potatoes to a serving dish.

3 Top with capers, parsley, and lemon peel. Drizzle with remaining olive oil. Squeeze lemon juice over potatoes before serving.

MAKE-AHEAD DIRECTIONS: Prepare as above through Step 2, except transfer mashed potato mixture to a storage container; cover and chill for up to 24 hours. To serve, transfer potato mixture to a large saucepan; heat through. Transfer to serving dish and top with capers, parsley, lemon peel, and olive oil. Squeeze lemon juice over potatoes before serving.

Roasted Cauliflower with Cranberries

Drizzle the balsamic-honey mixture over the roasted cauliflower while it's in the baking pan, then toss before transferring to the serving bowl.

SERVINGS 8 (1 cup each)
CARB. PER SERVING 21 g
PREP 15 minutes
ROAST 30 minutes
COOK 10 minutes

2   medium heads cauliflower (1½ to 2 pounds each), broken into large florets (8 cups)

1   large yellow or red onion, cut into wedges (2 cups)

3   tablespoons olive oil

¼   teaspoon kosher salt

1½ cups fresh or frozen cranberries

¼   cup balsamic vinegar

¼   cup honey

¼   teaspoon kosher salt

¼   teaspoon freshly cracked black pepper

1   tablespoon snipped fresh mint

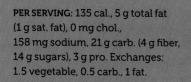

PER SERVING: 135 cal., 5 g total fat (1 g sat. fat), 0 mg chol., 158 mg sodium, 21 g carb. (4 g fiber, 14 g sugars), 3 g pro. Exchanges: 1.5 vegetable, 0.5 carb., 1 fat.

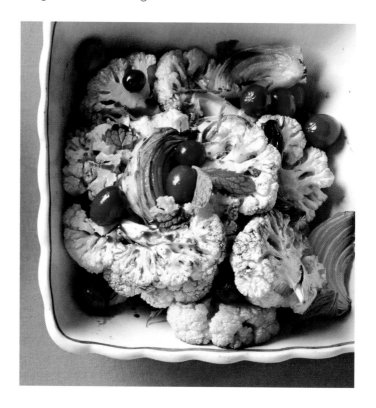

1 Preheat oven to 450ºF. Place cauliflower and onion in a shallow baking pan. Drizzle with olive oil and sprinkle with the ¼ teaspoon salt. Stir to coat. Spread in an even layer. Roast, uncovered, about 30 minutes or until cauliflower and onion are tender, stirring in cranberries halfway through roasting.

2 Meanwhile, in a small saucepan whisk together balsamic vinegar, honey, the remaining ¼ teaspoon salt, and pepper. Simmer, uncovered, until sightly thickened, about 10 minutes. Pour balsamic mixture over roasted cauliflower mixture; toss to coat. Transfer mixture to a serving dish. Sprinkle with mint.

Fresh Cranberry-Citrus Relish

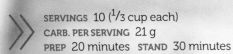

SERVINGS 10 (1/3 cup each)
CARB. PER SERVING 21 g
PREP 20 minutes **STAND** 30 minutes

1 medium seedless orange
1 medium lemon
1 medium apple
1/2 cup sugar*
4 cups fresh or frozen cranberries

PER SERVING: 77 cal., 0 g total fat,
0 mg chol., 1 mg sodium, 21 g carb.
(3 g fiber, 15 g sugars), 0 g pro.
Exchanges: 0.5 fruit, 0.5 carb..

1 Finely shred the peel from orange and lemon; set aside. Remove the remaining peel with a sharp knife and discard. Cut orange and lemon into wedges; discard any seeds. Core apple and cut into chunks.

2 Place fruit in a food processor. Add sugar. Cover and process with several on/off turns until coarsely chopped. Add cranberries. Cover and process with on/off turns until chopped. Transfer mixture to a bowl. Add reserved finely shredded orange and lemon peel; stir to combine.

3 Cover and let stand at room temperature for 30 to 45 minutes before serving, stirring occasionally.

*SUGAR SUBSTITUTE: We do not recommend using a sugar substitute for this recipe.

MAKE-AHEAD DIRECTIONS: Prepare relish. Cover and store in the refrigerator for up to 5 days.

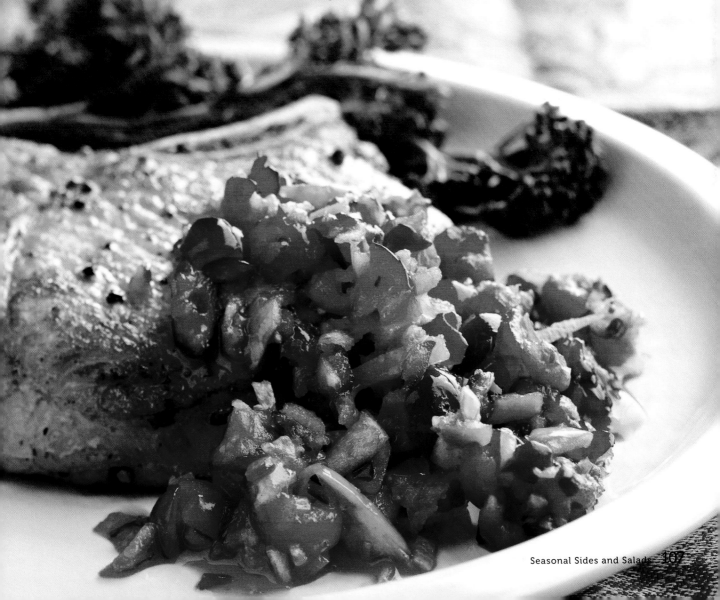

Broccoli-Cranberry Salad with Ginger-Honey Dressing

A sweet dressing, dried cranberries, and roasted pistachios put a holiday twist on traditional broccoli salad (AKA trees and raisins).

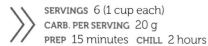

SERVINGS 6 (1 cup each)
CARB. PER SERVING 20 g
PREP 15 minutes   CHILL 2 hours

4 cups small fresh broccoli florets
¾ cup packaged fresh julienned carrots
½ cup thinly sliced celery (1 stalk)
½ cup thinly sliced green onions (4)
⅓ cup dried cranberries
¼ cup plain low-fat yogurt
2 tablespoons honey
1 tablespoon rice vinegar
1 tablespoon sesame oil or canola oil
1 teaspoon grated fresh ginger or ½ teaspoon ground ginger
¼ teaspoon salt
¼ teaspoon crushed red pepper (optional)
⅓ cup chopped roasted shelled pistachio nuts or toasted chopped almonds

1 | In a large bowl combine broccoli, carrots, celery, green onions, and cranberries.

2 | For dressing, in a small bowl combine yogurt, honey, vinegar, oil, ginger, salt, and crushed red pepper (if using). Drizzle dressing over broccoli mixture; stir until well combined.

3 | Cover and chill for 2 to 4 hours. Just before serving, stir in nuts.

PER SERVING: 137 cal., 6 g total fat (1 g sat. fat), 1 mg chol., 167 mg sodium, 20 g carb. (3 g fiber, 13 g sugars), 4 g pro. Exchanges: 1 vegetable, 1 carb., 1 fat.

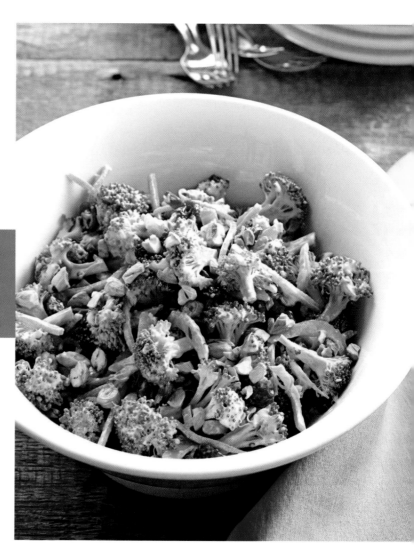

Fruited Multigrain Pilaf

There's no need to watch this pot—load the slow cooker and let it cook.

SERVINGS 12 (³/₄ cup each)
CARB. PER SERVING 31 g
PREP 20 minutes **SLOW COOK** 6 to 7 hours (low) or 3¹/₂ to 4 hours (high)

- ²/₃ cup uncooked wheat berries
- ¹/₂ cup uncooked pearled farro or regular barley
- ¹/₂ cup uncooked wild rice
- 4 cups unsalted chicken stock or vegetable stock
- 12 ounces sweet potato, peeled and chopped (2¹/₃ cups)
- ²/₃ cup dried cranberries
- ¹/₂ cup sliced celery (1 stalk)
- 1 tablespoon butter
- 2 cloves garlic, minced
- ¹/₂ teaspoon salt
- ¹/₄ teaspoon black pepper
- 1¹/₃ cups chopped red cooking apples, such as Rome or Jonathan (2 medium)
- ¹/₂ cup chopped, toasted walnuts
- ¹/₂ cup sliced green onions (4)
- 1 tablespoon snipped fresh thyme
- Fresh thyme sprigs (optional)

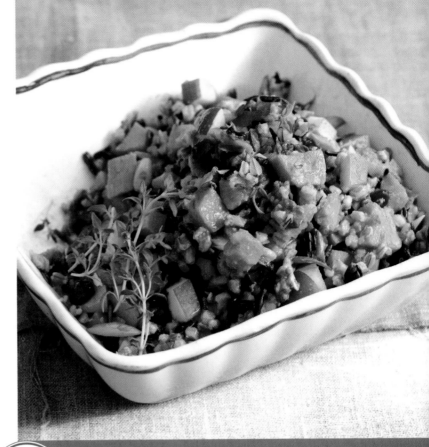

6 grams pro.

PER SERVING: 184 cal., 5 g total fat (1 g sat. fat), 3 mg chol., 177 mg sodium, 31 g carb. (4 g fiber, 7 g sugars), 6 g pro. Exchanges: 0.5 fruit, 1.5 starch, 0.5 fat.

1 Rinse and drain wheat berries, barley (if using), and wild rice. In a 3¹/₂- or 4-quart slow cooker stir together wheat berries, farro or barley, wild rice, stock, sweet potato, cranberries, celery, butter, garlic, salt, and pepper.

2 Cover and cook on low-heat setting for 6 to 7 hours or on high-heat setting for 3¹/₂ to 4 hours. Just before serving, stir in the apples, walnuts, green onions, and snipped thyme. Transfer to a serving dish. If desired, garnish with thyme sprigs.

QUICK TIP
Use a fine-mesh sieve to hold the wheat berries, barley (if using), and wild rice while rinsing. Stir or gently toss so all of the grains get equally rinsed.

Wild Rice and Bread Stuffing with Bacon

Thanks to the can of condensed cream of mushroom or chicken soup, this casserole has a creamier finish than classic stuffing.

SERVINGS 8 (½ cup each)
CARB. PER SERVING 21 g
PREP 30 minutes **COOK** 50 minutes **BAKE** 30 minutes

2 cups thinly sliced fresh button or cremini mushrooms

1 cup thinly sliced celery (2 stalks)

1 cup chopped onion (1 large)

¾ cup chopped red sweet pepper (1 medium)

4 slices lower-sodium, less-fat bacon, chopped

4 cloves garlic, minced

½ cup uncooked wild rice

2 cups water

¼ cup dried tomatoes (not oil-packed), finely snipped

1½ teaspoons dried thyme, crushed

1 10.75-ounce can reduced-fat, reduced-sodium condensed cream of mushroom or cream of chicken soup

4 slices reduced-calorie wheat or oatmeal bread, cut into ½-inch cubes and dried*

Water

Nonstick cooking spray

¼ cup snipped fresh Italian (flat-leaf) parsley or 2 tablespoons snipped fresh chives

1 In a 4-quart pot cook mushrooms, celery, onion, sweet pepper, and bacon over medium heat for 6 to 8 minutes or until vegetables are tender, stirring occasionally. Stir in garlic. Transfer vegetable mixture to a medium bowl; set aside.

2 Meanwhile, rinse wild rice with cold water. Add rice and the 2 cups water to the same pot used to cook vegetable mixture. Bring to boiling; reduce heat. Simmer, covered, for 40 minutes. Stir in tomatoes and thyme. Cover and cook for 5 to 10 minutes more or until rice is tender. Remove from the heat.

3 Preheat oven to 325°F. Add condensed soup to the rice mixture; stir until well combined. Stir in vegetable mixture. Add bread cubes; toss to combine. Add just enough additional water to moisten, tossing to combine. Lightly coat a 1½- or 2-quart casserole with cooking spray. Spoon stuffing mixture into casserole.

4 Bake, covered, for 25 minutes. Uncover and bake for 5 to 10 minutes more or until heated through. Sprinkle with parsley before serving.

*TEST KITCHEN TIP: To make dry bread cubes, preheat oven to 300°F. Spread cubes in a 15×10×1-inch baking pan. Bake for 10 to 15 minutes or until cubes are dry, stirring twice; cool. (Cubes will continue to dry and crisp as they cool.) Or let bread cubes stand, loosely covered, at room temperature for 8 to 12 hours.

21 grams carb

PER SERVING: 138 cal., 4 g total fat (1 g sat. fat), 5 mg chol., 223 mg sodium, 21 g carb. (4 g fiber, 4 g sugars), 6 g pro. Exchanges: 1 vegetable, 1 starch, 0.5 fat.

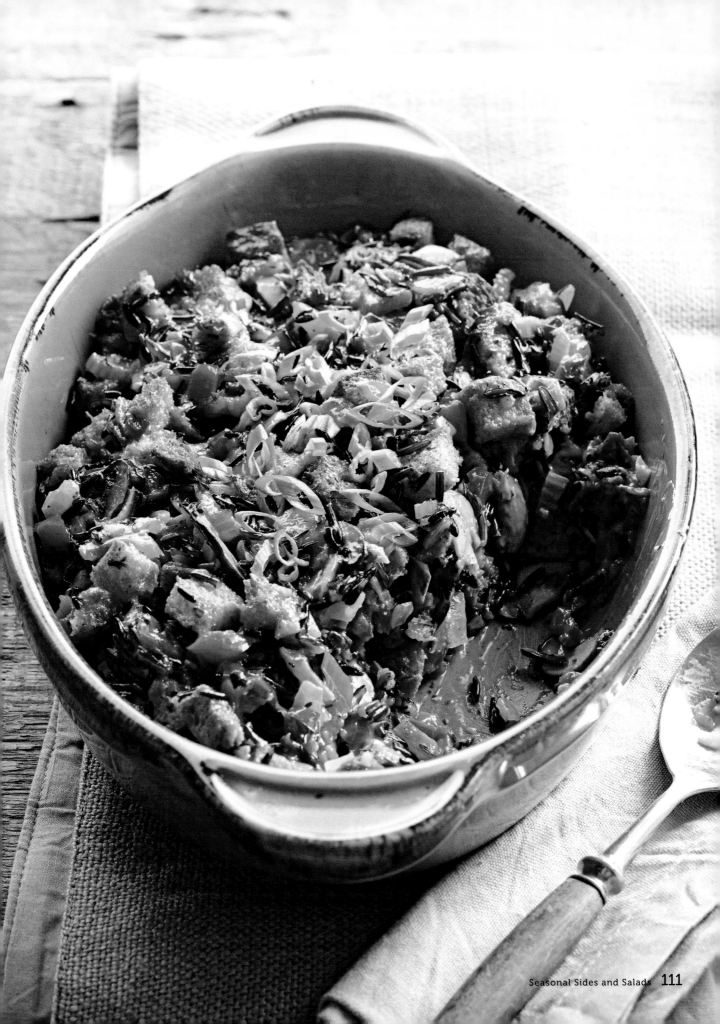

Crunchy Kale Salad with Creamy Tomato-Garlic Dressing

There will be extra dressing, so store it in an airtight container in the refrigerator for up 3 days and stir before using.

» SERVINGS 6 (³/4 cup salad and 1 tablespoon dressing each)
CARB. PER SERVING 9 g
START TO FINISH 45 minutes

1 recipe Creamy Tomato-Garlic Dressing

6 cups torn, trimmed fresh kale

2 teaspoons olive oil

¹/4 teaspoon salt

1 cup thin bite-size strips red, yellow, and/or orange sweet pepper

6 teaspoons slivered almonds, toasted and chopped

1 Prepare Creamy Tomato-Garlic Dressing. For salad, in a large bowl combine kale, olive oil, and salt. Using clean hands, rub and knead the oil and salt into the kale for about 2 minutes or until kale is softened and the volume is nearly half. Divide salad among six serving plates. Top with sweet pepper strips and almonds. Drizzle each salad with 1 tablespoon of the dressing. Store remaining dressing in an airtight container in the refrigerator for up to 1 week. Use on steamed or grilled vegetables or other salads.

CREAMY TOMATO-GARLIC DRESSING: Preheat oven to 425°F. Peel away the dry outer layers of skin from 1 head of garlic, leaving skins and cloves intact. Cut off the pointed top portion (about ¹/4 inch), leaving bulb intact but exposing the individual cloves. Place the garlic head, cut side up, in a custard cup. Drizzle with ¹/2 teaspoon olive oil. Cover with foil and bake for 25 to 35 minutes or until cloves feel soft when pressed. Set aside just until cool enough to handle. Meanwhile, in a small bowl combine ¹/4 cup boiling water and 3 tablespoons snipped dried tomatoes (not oil-packed). Cover and let stand for 10 minutes. Pour undrained tomato mixture into a blender. Squeeze garlic cloves from the peels and add to blender. Add 2¹/2 teaspoons olive oil, ²/3 cup buttermilk, 1 teaspoon finely shredded lemon peel, 2 tablespoons lemon juice, ¹/8 teaspoon salt, and ¹/8 teaspoon black pepper. Cover and blend until smooth, scraping sides of blender as necessary.

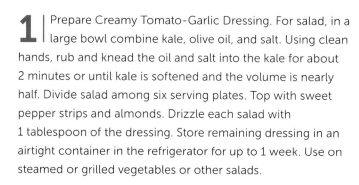

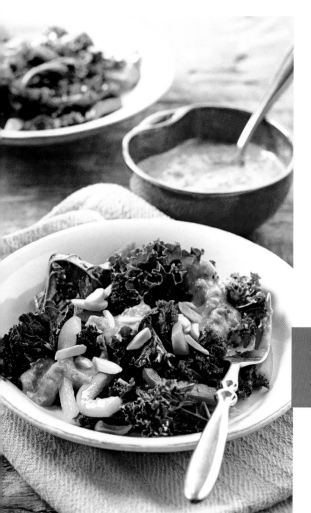

PER SERVING: 80 cal., 4 g total fat (1 g sat. fat), 0 mg chol., 148 mg sodium, 9 g carb. (2 g fiber, 3 g sugars), 4 g pro. Exchanges: 1.5 vegetable, 1 fat.

4 grams pro.

Persimmon and Blue Cheese Spinach Salad

Persimmons are available October through January. They are ripe and ready to use when they yield to gentle pressure when lightly squeezed.

SERVINGS 6 (1 cup greens, $1/3$ of a persimmon, 1 tablespoon cheese, and $1^1/2$ teaspoon nuts each)
CARB. PER SERVING 6 g
PREP 25 minutes CHILL 4 hours

- $1/3$ cup red wine vinegar
- 1 medium shallot, very thinly sliced
- 2 tablespoons snipped fresh basil
- 2 tablespoons olive oil
- 1 teaspoon Dijon-style mustard
- $1/8$ teaspoon salt
- Dash black pepper
- 4 cups packaged fresh baby spinach
- 1 head radicchio, trimmed, cored, and coarsely chopped (about 3 cups)
- 2 medium ripe Fuyu persimmons or red tomatoes, cored and cut into thin wedges
- 6 tablespoons crumbled reduced-fat blue cheese
- 3 tablespoons chopped, toasted hazelnuts or walnuts

PER SERVING: 112 cal., 8 g total fat (2 g sat. fat), 4 mg chol., 198 mg sodium, 6 g carb. (2 g fiber, 1 g sugars), 4 g pro. Exchanges: 1 vegetable, 1.5 fat.

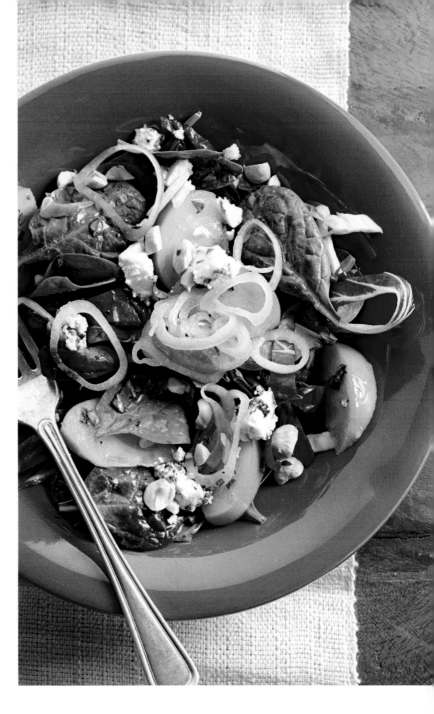

1 In a small bowl combine vinegar and shallot. Cover and chill for at least 4 hours or up to 24 hours, stirring occasionally.

2 Using a slotted spoon, transfer shallots to another small bowl; set aside. For vinaigrette, add basil, oil, mustard, salt, and pepper to vinegar. Whisk until well combined.

3 In a large bowl combine spinach and radicchio. Drizzle with half the vinaigrette. Toss gently to coat. Divide spinach mixture among six serving plates. Top with persimmon wedges, blue cheese, and hazelnuts. Drizzle evenly with remaining vinaigrette. Top with shallot slices.

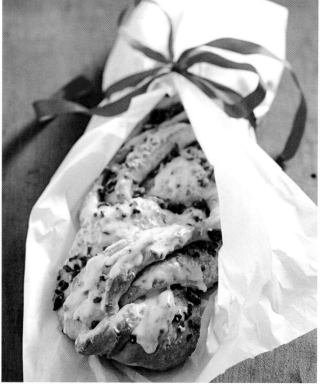

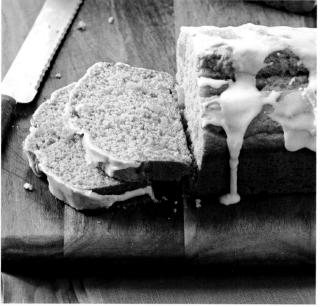

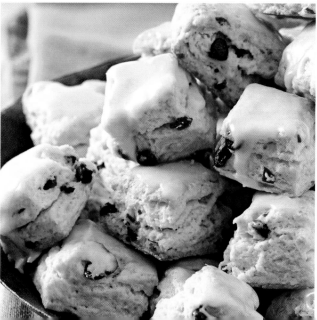

fresh-baked
breads

Whether it's a fruit-studded quick loaf, a rich and flaky scone,

or an icing-topped yeasted twist, homemade bread is hard to

resist—especially at the holidays. This season grace the table

with one or more of these spectacular baked goods. Each one is

wholesomely nutritious and ultimately delicious.

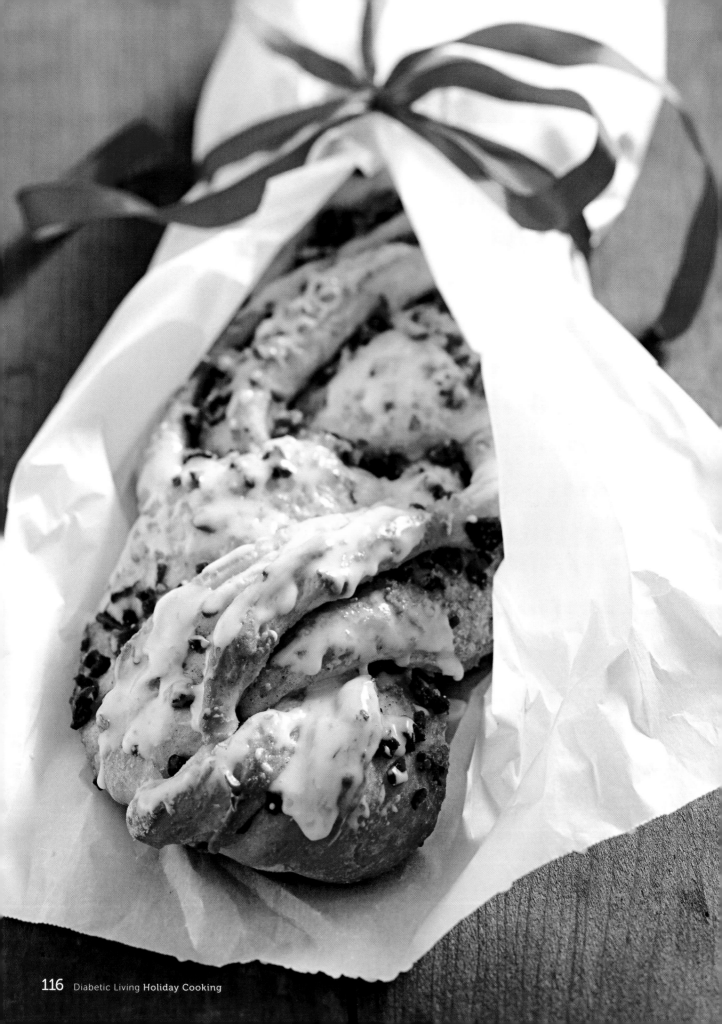

Cranberry Twist Bread

Stash the extra fresh cranberries in a freezer container or bag and freeze up to 1 year for another use.

SERVINGS 16 (1 slice each)
CARB. PER SERVING 21 g or 18 g
PREP 30 minutes **RISE** 1 hour 30 minutes **STAND** 10 minutes **BAKE** 25 minutes

2½ to 3 cups flour

1 package active dry yeast

¾ cup fat-free milk

⅓ cup granulated sugar*

2 tablespoons butter or margarine

½ teaspoon salt

1 egg

½ cup finely chopped cranberries

2 tablespoons finely chopped pecans

1½ teaspoons finely shredded orange peel

½ teaspoon pumpkin pie spice or apple pie spice

1½ teaspoons butter or margarine, melted

1 recipe Orange Icing (optional)

PER SERVING: 121 cal., 3 g total fat (1 g sat. fat), 17 mg chol., 99 mg sodium, 21 g carb. (1 g fiber, 5 g sugars), 3 g pro. Exchanges: 1 starch, 0.5 carb., 0.5 fat.

PER SERVING WITH SUBSTITUTE: Same as above, except 115 cal., 98 mg sodium, 18 g carb. (3 g sugars). Exchanges: 0 carb.

1 | In a large bowl stir together 1 cup of the flour and the yeast; set aside. In a small saucepan heat and stir milk, 2 tablespoons of the granulated sugar, the 2 tablespoons butter, and salt until warm (120°F to 130°F). Add milk mixture to flour mixture; add egg. Beat with an electric mixer on low to medium speed for 30 seconds, scraping bowl. Beat on high speed for 3 minutes. Stir in as much of the remaining flour as you can.

2 | Turn dough out onto a floured surface. Knead in enough remaining flour to make a soft dough that is smooth and elastic (3 to 5 minutes total). Shape dough into a ball. Place in a lightly greased bowl; turn once to grease surface of dough. Cover and let rise in a warm place until double in size (1 to 1½ hours).

3 | For filling, in a small bowl combine cranberries, remaining sugar, the pecans, orange peel, and spice; set aside.

4 | Punch down dough. Turn out onto lightly floured surface. Cover; let rest 10 minutes. Grease a baking sheet. Roll dough into a 14×10-inch rectangle. Brush with the 1½ teaspoons melted butter. Sprinkle filling over dough. Starting from a long side, roll dough into a spiral. Seal seam. Place seam side down and cut roll in half lengthwise. Place cut sides up, side by side, on prepared baking sheet. Loosely twist halves together, keeping cut sides up. Pinch ends to seal. Cover; let rise in a warm place until nearly double in size (about 30 minutes).

5 | Preheat oven to 375°F. Bake about 25 minutes or until golden brown (if necessary, cover loosely with foil the last 10 minutes to prevent overbrowning). Remove from baking sheet; cool on a wire rack. If desired, drizzle with Orange Icing.

ORANGE ICING: In a medium bowl combine 1½ cups powdered sugar,* 1 teaspoon finely shredded orange peel, and 2 to 3 tablespoons orange juice to make icing a drizzling consistency.

*SUGAR SUBSTITUTES: Choose Splenda Sugar Blend for Baking to substitute for the granulated sugar. Follow package directions to use product equivalent to ⅓ cup granulated sugar. We do not recommend using a sugar substitute for the powdered sugar.

No-Knead Bread

This artisan-textured bread is mixed in the same saucepan that it is baked in, making cleanup quite simple.

SERVINGS 12 (1 slice each)
CARB. PER SERVING 24 g or 23 g
PREP 25 minutes
STAND 1 hour 30 minutes
CHILL overnight **BAKE** 40 minutes

1½ cups warm water (105°F to 115°F)

1 teaspoon active dry yeast

2¾ cups bread flour

2 tablespoons sugar*

2 tablespoons olive oil

1¼ teaspoons salt

1 In a 2-quart oven-going, nonstick saucepan** stir together the warm water and yeast until yeast is dissolved. Stir in flour, sugar, oil, and salt until combined. Cover with lid; let stand in a warm place for 1 hour. Stir down. Cover and chill overnight.

2 Before baking, let dough stand, uncovered, at room temperature for 30 minutes. Preheat oven to 425°F. Bake in the saucepan, uncovered, about 40 minutes or until top is golden, bread sounds hollow when lightly tapped, and an instant-read thermometer inserted in the center registers 200°F. If necessary to prevent overbrowning, cover loosely with foil for the last 15 minutes of baking.

3 Immediately loosen sides and remove bread from saucepan. Transfer to a wire rack. Cool. Cut into 12 slices.

*SUGAR SUBSTITUTES: Choose from Splenda Sugar Blend for Baking or Equal Sugar Lite. Follow package directions to use product amount equivalent to 2 tablespoons sugar.

**TEST KITCHEN TIP: For a traditional loaf-shape bread, use an 8×4×2-inch loaf pan instead of the saucepan. Line the loaf pan with parchment paper. Mix the dough in a large bowl and transfer to the prepared loaf pan; cover with greased or nonstick foil during standing and chilling in Step 1. Bake about 35 minutes or until top is golden, bread sounds hollow when lightly tapped, and an instant-read thermometer inserted in the center registers 200°F.

CINNAMON-RAISIN BREAD: Prepare as directed, except stir in ½ cup raisins and ½ teaspoon ground cinnamon with the flour. Cover loosely with foil for the last 15 minutes of baking.

PER SERVING (WITH SUGAR): Same as above, except 152 cal., 29 g carb. (6 g sugars). Exchanges: 0.5 carb.

PER SERVING: 133 cal., 3 g total fat (0 g sat. fat), 0 mg chol., 207 mg sodium, 24 g carb. (1 g fiber, 2 g sugars), 3 g pro. Exchanges: 1.5 starch.

PER SERVING WITH SUBSTITUTE: Same as above, except 130 cal., 23 g carb. (1 g sugars).

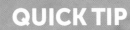

QUICK TIP

This raisin-studded loaf is perfect for toasting. Slice the loaf and store it in a freezer bag in the freezer. You can then pull out one slice at a time for toasting and eating.

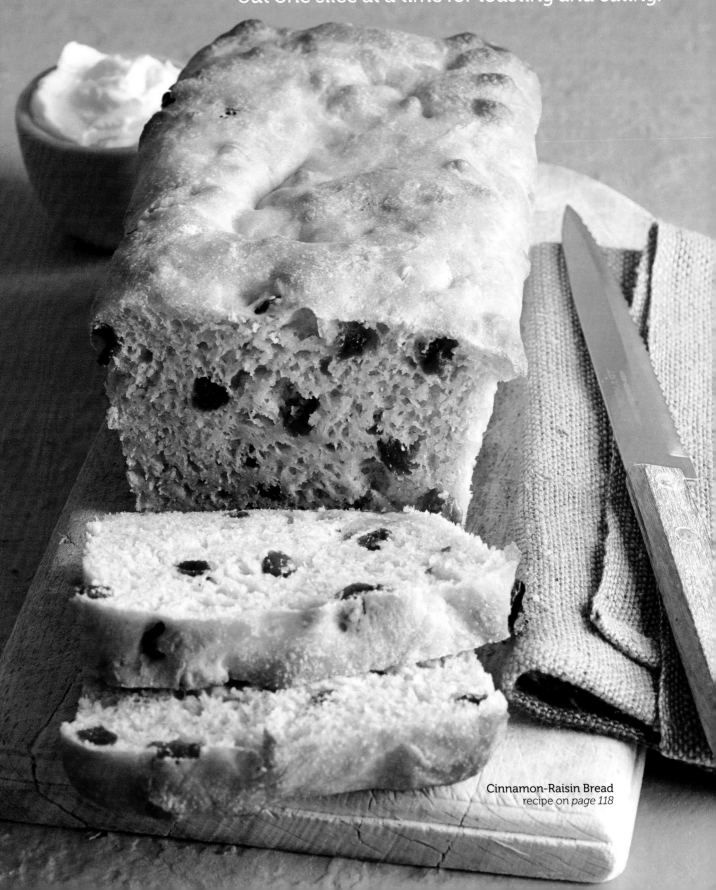

Cinnamon-Raisin Bread
recipe on *page 118*

Slow Cooker Herb and Garlic Peasant Bread

That's right! This hearty yeast bread is formulated to cook in a 6-quart slow cooker, but a few minutes under the broiler give it a golden brown finish.

SERVINGS 16 (1 slice each)
CARB. PER SERVING 26 g or 25 g
PREP 25 minutes **STAND** 2 hours 40 minutes **SLOW COOK** $2^{1}/4$ to $2^{1}/2$ hours (high) **BROIL** 3 minutes

$1^{1}/4$ cups warm water (105°F to 115°F)

1 tablespoon active dry yeast

1 teaspoon sugar*

$^{1}/4$ cup warm fat-free milk (105°F to 115°F)

2 cloves garlic, minced

$^{1}/2$ cup plain low-fat yogurt (room temperature)

1 tablespoon snipped fresh thyme, basil, or rosemary

$1^{1}/2$ teaspoons salt

$3^{3}/4$ cups all-purpose flour

$^{1}/4$ cup whole wheat flour

Nonstick cooking spray

1 tablespoon yellow cornmeal

PER SERVING: 125 cal., 1 g total fat (0 g sat. fat), 1 mg chol., 227 mg sodium, 26 g carb. (1 g fiber, 1 g sugars), 4 g pro. Exchanges: 1.5 starch.

PER SERVING WITH SUBSTITUTE: Same as above, except 25 g carb.

1 In an extra-large bowl stir together the warm water, yeast, and sugar; let stand about 10 minutes or until mixture is foamy.

2 In a small bowl stir together warm milk and garlic. Stir milk mixture, yogurt, thyme, and salt into yeast mixture. In a medium bowl stir together all-purpose flour and whole wheat flour. Add $2^{1}/2$ cups of the flour mixture to the yeast mixture; stir just until combined. Cover bowl with plastic wrap; let stand at room temperature for 2 hours. Set remaining flour mixture aside.

3 Stir $1^{1}/4$ cups of the remaining flour mixture into dough. Sprinkle a work surface with remaining $^{1}/4$ cup flour mixture; turn dough out onto the floured surface. Knead for 2 to 3 minutes (dough will be sticky; flour hands as needed). Cover dough on work surface; let stand at room temperature for 30 minutes.

4 Lightly coat the inside of a 6-quart slow cooker with cooking spray. Line the bottom of the cooker with parchment paper; coat paper with cooking spray and sprinkle evenly with cornmeal. Dust top of dough lightly with additional all-purpose flour; shape dough into a "loose" ball using well-floured hands. Place dough in the center of the prepared cooker.

5 Cover and cook on high-heat setting for $2^{1}/4$ to $2^{1}/2$ hours or until an instant-read thermometer inserted near the center registers 200°F. If possible, turn the crockery liner a half-turn halfway through cooking (do not lift the lid).

6 Preheat broiler. Remove loaf from cooker by carefully inverting onto a wire rack; if necessary, peel off parchment paper. Turn loaf upright and place on an ungreased baking sheet. Broil 5 to 6 inches from the heat for 3 to 4 minutes or until top of loaf is light brown and surface is no longer moist. Transfer to a wire rack. Cool. Cut into 16 slices.

*SUGAR SUBSTITUTE: Choose Splenda Sugar Blend for Baking. Follow package directions to use product equivalent to 1 teaspoon sugar.

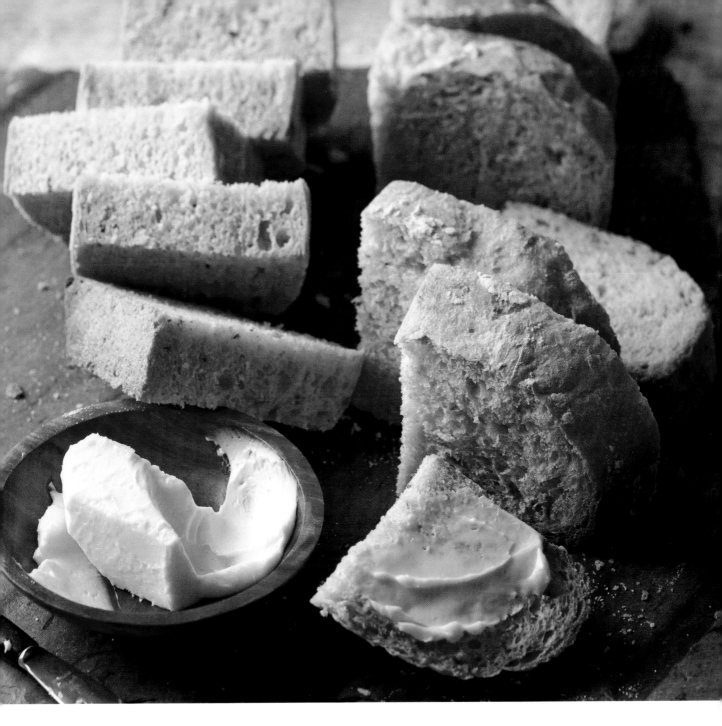

SLOW COOKER ONION AND DILL PEASANT BREAD:
Prepare as directed in Step 1. Prepare
Step 2, except omit garlic and herb. Stir
1 tablespoon dill seeds and 1 tablespoon
minced dried onion in with the yeast mixture,
yogurt, warm milk, and salt. Continue as
directed through Step 5. If desired, before
broiling, brush the top of the loaf with
1 tablespoon melted butter and sprinkle with
$1/4$ to $1/2$ teaspoon kosher or coarse salt.

PER SERVING (WITH SUGAR): Same as herb-garlic
bread, except 126 cal.

SLOW COOKER FENNEL AND BLACK PEPPER PEASANT
BREAD: Prepare as directed in Step 1. Prepare
Step 2, except omit garlic and herb. Stir
2 teaspoons fennel seeds and $1/2$ teaspoon
freshly ground black pepper in with the yeast
mixture, yogurt, warm milk, and salt. Continue
as directed.

PER SERVING (WITH SUGAR): Same as herb-garlic
bread, except 126 cal.

Overnight Refrigerator Rolls

Immediately remove the baked rolls from the pan and place on a cooling rack. If the rolls are left in the pan, the bottoms will get soggy.

SERVINGS 24 (1 roll each)
CARB. PER SERVING 19 g or 17 g
PREP 35 minutes **CHILL** overnight **RISE** 45 minutes **BAKE** 12 minutes

1¼ cups warm water (105°F to 115°F)

1 package active dry yeast

4 to 4¼ cups flour

⅓ cup sugar*

⅓ cup butter, melted, or vegetable oil

1 egg

1 teaspoon salt

Nonstick cooking spray

2 tablespoons butter, melted (optional)

PER SERVING: 114 cal., 3 g total fat (2 g sat. fat), 15 mg chol., 123 mg sodium, 19 g carb. (1 g fiber, 3 g sugars), 3 g pro. Exchanges: 1 starch, 0.5 fat.

PER SERVING WITH SUBSTITUTE: Same as above, except 109 cal., 17 g carb. (1 g sugars).

1 In a large mixing bowl combine the warm water and yeast; stir to dissolve yeast. Add 1½ cups of the flour, the sugar, ⅓ cup melted butter, egg, and salt. Beat with an electric mixer on low speed for 1 minute, scraping sides of bowl constantly. Using a wooden spoon, stir in enough of the remaining flour to make a soft dough that just starts to pull away from sides of bowl (dough will be slightly sticky).

2 Coat the inside of a 3-quart covered container with cooking spray. Place dough in container; turn once to grease surface of dough. Cover and chill overnight.

3 Punch dough down. Turn dough out onto a lightly floured surface. Divide dough in half. Cover and let rest for 10 minutes. Meanwhile, lightly grease a 13×9×2-inch baking pan or baking sheets.

4 Shape dough into 24 balls or desired rolls (be careful not to overwork dough; it becomes stickier the more you work with it) and place in the prepared baking pan or 2 to 3 inches apart on the prepared baking sheets. Cover and let rise in a warm place until nearly double in size (about 45 minutes).

5 Preheat oven to 375°F. Bake for 12 to 15 minutes for individual rolls, about 20 minutes for pan rolls, or until golden. Immediately remove rolls from pans. If desired, brush tops of rolls with the 2 tablespoons melted butter. Serve warm.

*SUGAR SUBSTITUTES: Choose from Splenda Sugar Blend for Baking or C&H Light Sugar & Stevia Blend. Follow package directions to use product amount equivalent to ⅓ cup sugar.

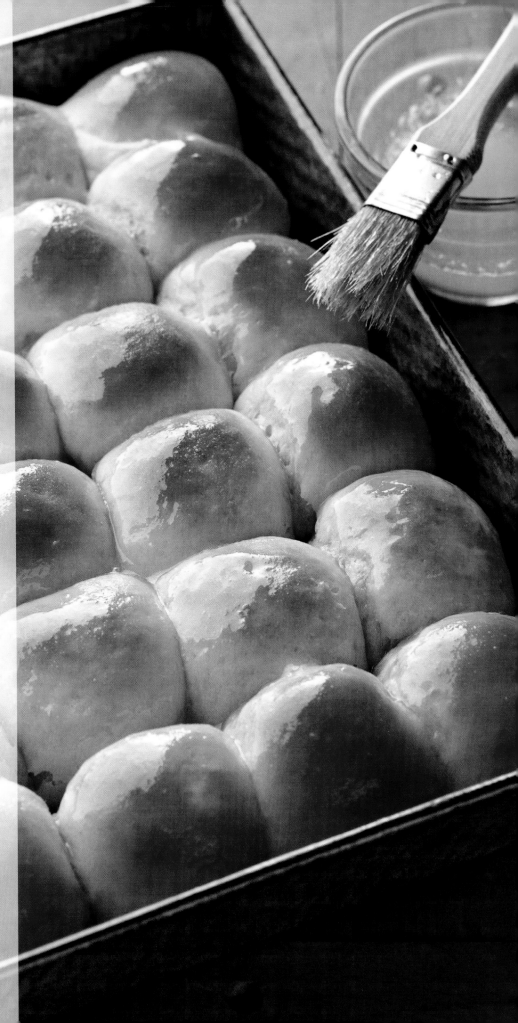

PARMESAN-HERB ROSETTES: Prepare as directed through Step 3, except add ½ teaspoon dried rosemary, crushed, or 1 teaspoon dried thyme or oregano, crushed, to the dough during Step 1. Divide each dough half into 16 pieces. On a lightly floured surface roll each piece into a 12-inch rope. Tie each rope in a loose knot, leaving two long ends. Tuck top end under the knot and bottom end into the top center. Brush with melted butter and sprinkle with grated Parmesan cheese. Place 2 to 3 inches apart on the prepared baking sheets. Continue as directed. Makes 32 rolls.

PER SERVING: Same as basic recipe, except 93 cal., 13 mg chol., 106 mg sodium, 14 g carb. (0 g fiber, 2 g sugars), 2 g pro.

SALT-AND-PEPPER PARKER HOUSE ROLLS: Prepare as directed through Step 3. On a lightly floured surface roll each dough half until ¼ inch thick. Cut dough with a floured 2½-inch round cutter. Using the dull edge of a table knife, make an off-center crease in each round. Fold each round along the crease; press the folded edge firmly. Place rolls, larger halves up, 2 to 3 inches apart on the prepared baking sheets. Brush with melted butter and sprinkle generously with kosher salt and freshly ground black pepper. Continue as directed. Makes 24 rolls.

PER SERVING: Same as basic recipe, except 122 cal., 4 g fat, 17 mg chol., 214 mg sodium.

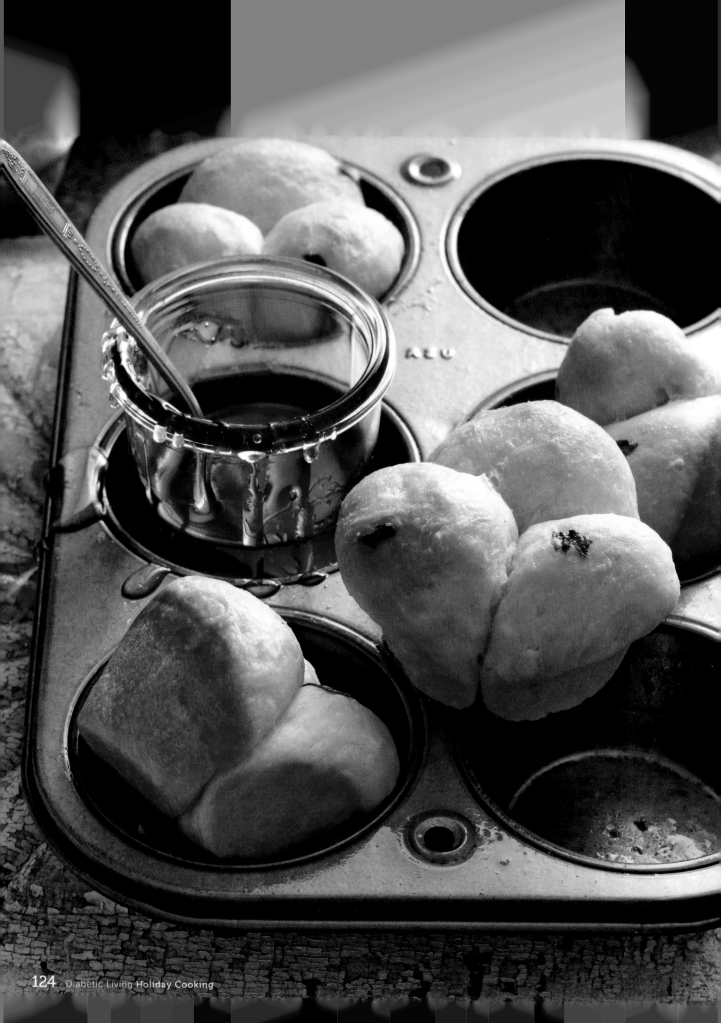

Buttermilk-Sage Cloverleaf Rolls

You can use sour milk instead of buttermilk. To make your own sour milk, pour 4$\frac{1}{2}$ teaspoons vinegar into a 2-cup glass measuring cup. Add milk to equal 1$\frac{1}{2}$ cups total. Let stand for 5 minutes.

SERVINGS 24 (1 roll each)
CARB. PER SERVING 20 g
PREP 45 minutes **RISE** 1 hour **BAKE** 15 minutes

$\frac{1}{2}$ cup unsalted butter, cut up

2 tablespoons snipped fresh sage leaves

3 tablespoons sugar*

1$\frac{1}{2}$ cups buttermilk

2 packages active dry yeast

$\frac{1}{2}$ cup warm water (105°F to 115°F)

4$\frac{1}{2}$ cups flour

2 teaspoons kosher salt

$\frac{1}{2}$ teaspoon baking soda

2 tablespoons butter, melted

PER SERVING: 142 cal., 5 g total fat (3 g sat. fat), 13 mg chol., 208 mg sodium, 20 g carb. (1 g fiber, 2 g sugars), 3 g pro. Exchanges: 1 starch, 1 fat.

PER SERVING WITH SUBSTITUTE: Same as above, except 140 cal.

1 Lightly grease twenty-four 2$\frac{1}{2}$-inch muffin cups; set aside. In a saucepan combine $\frac{1}{2}$ cup butter, 1 tablespoon of the sage, and 2 tablespoons of the sugar. Heat and stir over medium-high heat just until butter is melted. Stir in buttermilk and heat just until warmed (do not boil). Remove from heat; cool to room temperature.

2 In a small bowl combine the yeast and the remaining 1 tablespoon sugar. Stir in the warm water; let stand about 5 minutes or until yeast foams. Add the yeast mixture to the buttermilk mixture; stir to combine.

3 In a large bowl stir together the flour, salt, and baking soda. Add the buttermilk-yeast mixture. Stir to combine, forming a sticky dough. Loosely cover the bowl; let stand in a warm place until dough has risen slightly (about 30 minutes).

4 Turn dough out onto a lightly floured surface. Knead several times or until dough is easy to handle. Pinch off pieces of dough and form into 1-inch balls. To shape cloverleaf rolls, place three 1-inch balls in each prepared muffin cup. Loosely cover rolls with a clean cloth and let rise in a warm place until double in size (30 to 45 minutes).

5 Preheat oven to 375°F. In a small bowl combine 2 tablespoons melted butter and remaining 1 tablespoon sage. Uncover rolls. Brush lightly with melted butter mixture. Bake about 15 minutes or until golden brown. Remove rolls from muffin cups. Serve warm.

*SUGAR SUBSTITUTES: Choose from Splenda Sugar Blend for Baking or C&H Light Sugar and Stevia Blend. Follow package directions to use product amount equivalent to 3 tablespoons sugar.

MAKE-AHEAD DIRECTIONS: Place rolls in a freezer container; label and freeze for up to 1 month. Thaw completely. To reheat, wrap rolls in foil and place in a 350°F oven about 15 minutes or until heated through.

Easy Parmesan-Fennel Rolls

You don't need bread-baking experience to turn out these dinner rolls—start with frozen bread dough and choose one of three shapes.

SERVINGS 12 (1 roll each)
CARB. PER SERVING 18 g
PREP 25 minutes   **RISE** 30 minutes
BAKE 10 minutes

- 1   16-ounce loaf frozen white or wheat bread dough
- 1   tablespoon grated Parmesan cheese
- 2   teaspoons yellow cornmeal
- ½   teaspoon fennel seeds
- 2   tablespoons butter, melted

1 Thaw dough according to package directions. Grease a large baking sheet; set aside. In a small bowl stir together Parmesan cheese, cornmeal, and fennel seeds; set aside.

2 Divide dough into 12 equal pieces. Shape dough using one of the shaping options below. Cover with waxed paper and let rise in a warm place until nearly double in size (about 30 minutes). Gently brush with melted butter and sprinkle with cheese mixture.

3 Preheat oven to 375°F. Bake, uncovered, for 10 to 15 minutes or until golden. Transfer rolls to a wire rack. Cool slightly before serving.

HOT CROSS-STYLE ROLLS: Divide dough into 12 pieces. Gently shape each piece into a ball by pulling dough and pinching underneath. Place balls 2 to 3 inches apart on the prepared baking sheet. Using kitchen shears, cut two deep snips to form an "X" shape in the top of each bun. Continue as directed.

S-SHAPE ROLLS: Divide dough into 12 pieces. Roll each piece into a 10-inch-long rope. Place on the prepared baking sheet. Twist the ends of each rope in the opposite directions. Shape each twisted rope into an "S" shape. Continue as directed.

DINNER ROLL KNOTS: Divide dough into 12 pieces. Roll each piece into a 12-inch-long rope. Tie each rope into a loose knot, leaving two long ends. Tuck the top end of the rope under roll. Bring the bottom end up and tuck into center of roll. Place knots 2 to 3 inches apart on the prepared baking sheet. Continue as directed.

MAKE-AHEAD DIRECTIONS: Place rolls in an airtight container or resealable plastic bag; cover or seal. Store at room temperature for up to 3 days. To reheat, place rolls on a baking sheet and bake in a 350°F oven for 5 to 6 minutes or until warm.

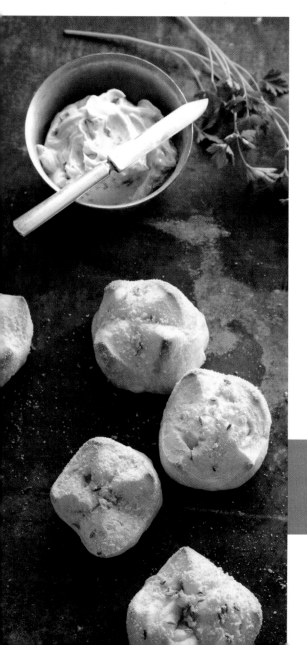

PER SERVING: 117 cal., 3 g total fat (1 g sat. fat), 5 mg chol., 194 mg sodium, 18 g carb. (0 g fiber, 1 g sugars), 2 g pro.
Exchanges: 1 starch, 0.5 fat.

Fig-Pistachio Baguette

Lightly coat the blade of a chef's knife with nonstick cooking spray before chopping the figs—this will keep them from sticking.

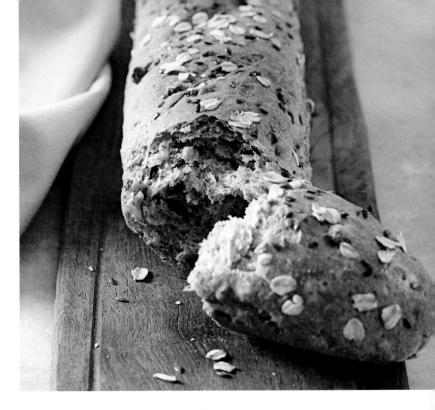

SERVINGS 16 (1 slice each)
CARB. PER SERVING 18 g
PREP 25 minutes **STAND** 6 hours
RISE 1 hour 30 minutes **BAKE** 15 minutes

- 2 to 2¼ cups all-purpose flour
- ½ cup warm water (105°F to 115°F)
- 1 teaspoon active dry yeast
- ½ cup warm water (105°F to 115°F)
- 1 teaspoon salt
- ½ cup oat flour
- ⅓ cup chopped pistachio nuts
- ¼ cup flaxseed meal
- ¼ cup chopped, stemmed dried figs
- 1 teaspoon finely shredded orange peel
- 1 tablespoon fat-free milk
- 2 tablespoons regular rolled oats or quick-cooking rolled oats
- 2 teaspoons flaxseed

PER SERVING: 106 cal., 2 g total fat (0 g sat. fat), 0 mg chol., 158 mg sodium, 18 g carb. (2 g fiber, 1 g sugars), 4 g pro. Exchanges: 1 starch, 0.5 fat.

1 | In a large bowl stir together ½ cup of the all-purpose flour, ½ cup warm water, and the yeast. Whisk lightly until smooth. Cover bowl loosely with plastic wrap. Let stand at room temperature for 6 to 12 hours to ferment.

2 | Gradually stir in remaining ½ cup warm water and the salt. Stir in oat flour, pistachios, flaxseed meal, figs, and orange peel. Stir in just enough of the remaining all-purpose flour to make a dough that pulls away from the sides of the bowl. Turn dough out onto a lightly floured surface. Knead in enough of the remaining all-purpose flour to make a soft dough that is smooth and elastic (3 to 5 minutes total).

3 | Place dough in a lightly greased bowl; turn once to grease surface of dough. Cover and let rise in a warm place until double in size (about 1 hour). Punch dough down. Let rest for 10 minutes.

4 | Lightly grease a baguette pan or large baking sheet; set aside. On a lightly floured surface gently roll dough to a 14-inch-long oval. Roll up from the long side, pinching dough to seal the seams. Place loaf, seam side down, in or on the prepared pan.

5 | Using a very sharp knife, make about five shallow slits across the top of the loaf. Brush top of loaf with the milk. Sprinkle top evenly with oats and flaxseed. Cover with plastic wrap and let rise in a warm place until nearly double in size (about 30 minutes).

6 | Preheat oven to 400°F. Bake for 15 to 20 minutes or until light brown. Transfer loaf to a wire rack; cool slightly or completely. Slice crosswise to serve.

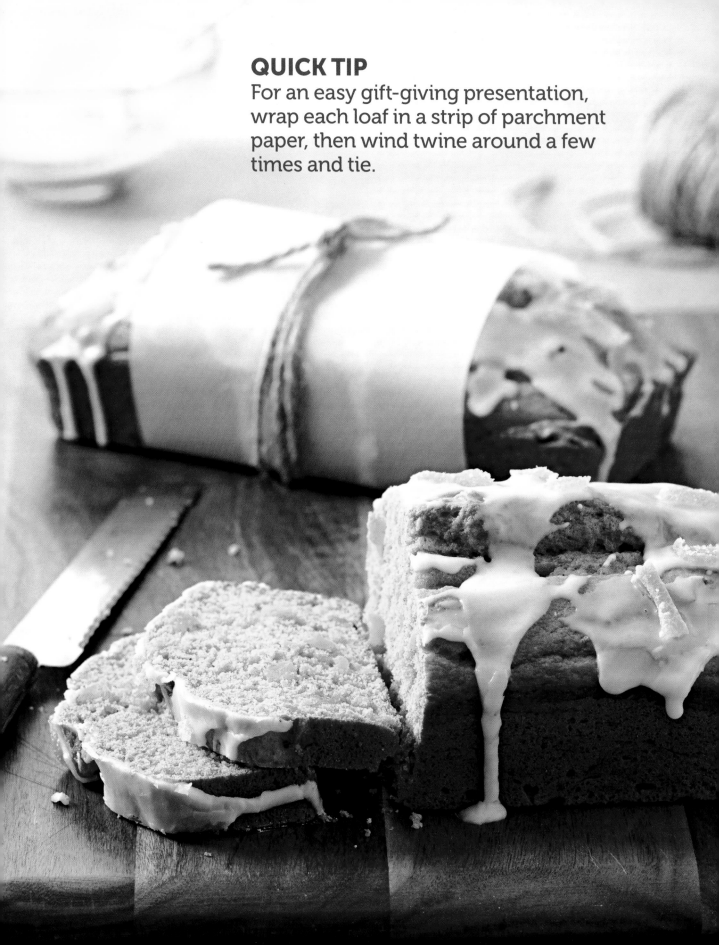

QUICK TIP
For an easy gift-giving presentation, wrap each loaf in a strip of parchment paper, then wind twine around a few times and tie.

Ginger-Apricot Pumpkin Loaves

There will be extra pumpkin. Instead of tossing it out, blend a little into a smoothie or swirl a bit into a bowl of hot breakfast cereal.

SERVINGS 24 (1 slice each)
CARB. PER SERVING 21 g
PREP 25 minutes **BAKE** 35 minutes **COOL** 10 minutes **STAND** overnight

1 cup all-purpose flour

1 cup whole wheat flour

3/4 cup granulated sugar*

1 tablespoon finely chopped crystallized ginger

2 1/2 teaspoons baking powder

1/2 teaspoon baking soda

1/2 teaspoon ground nutmeg

1/4 teaspoon salt

1 cup canned pumpkin

1/2 cup fat-free milk

2 eggs

1/3 cup shortening

1 cup finely snipped dried apricots or chopped pitted dates

1 recipe Spiced Glaze

Crystallized ginger, finely chopped (optional)

1 Preheat oven to 350°F. Lightly grease the bottoms and halfway up the sides of four 6×3 1/4×2-inch loaf pans or 1/2 inch up the sides of two 8×4×2-inch loaf pans; set aside.

2 In a large mixing bowl stir together all-purpose flour, whole wheat flour, granulated sugar, the 1 tablespoon ginger, the baking powder, baking soda, nutmeg, and salt. Add pumpkin, milk, eggs, and shortening. Beat with an electric mixer on low to medium speed for 30 seconds. Beat on high speed for 2 minutes, scraping sides of bowl occasionally. Stir in apricots. Spoon the batter evenly into prepared pans.

3 Bake about 30 minutes for 6×3 1/4×2-inch pans (about 35 minutes for 8×4×2-inch pans) or until a wooden toothpick inserted near centers comes out clean. Cool in pans on wire racks for 10 minutes. Remove from pans; cool completely on wire racks. Wrap and store overnight before slicing.

4 Before serving, drizzle with Spiced Glaze. If desired, sprinkle with additional chopped crystallized ginger. Let stand until glaze is set. Cut each small loaf into six slices or each large loaf into 12 slices.

SPICED GLAZE: In a small bowl stir together 2/3 cup powdered sugar* and 1/8 teaspoon ground ginger. Using 3 to 4 teaspoons water, stir in enough water, 1 teaspoon at a time, until glaze reaches drizzling consistency.

***SUGAR SUBSTITUTES:** We do not recommend using sugar substitutes for this recipe.

PER SERVING: 121 cal., 3 g total fat (1 g sat. fat), 16 mg chol., 111 mg sodium, 21 g carb. (1 g fiber, 12 g sugars), 2 g pro. Exchanges: 0.5 starch, 1 carb., 0.5 fat.

3 grams fat

Tangerine-Poppy Seed Quick Bread

Depending on the size, it may take two tangerines to squeeze enough juice for this citrus loaf. Oranges will work if tangerines are not available.

SERVINGS 16 (1 slice each)
CARB. PER SERVING 28 g or 20 g
PREP 25 minutes   **BAKE** 50 minutes   **COOL** 10 minutes
STAND overnight

2   cups flour
1   cup sugar*
2   teaspoons baking powder
½   teaspoon salt
1   cup fat-free milk
1   egg, lightly beaten
¼   cup vegetable oil
1   tablespoon finely shredded tangerine peel
2   tablespoons tangerine juice
1   tablespoon poppy seeds
2   tablespoons sugar*
2   tablespoons tangerine juice
1   tablespoon butter

1 | Preheat oven to 350°F. Grease the bottom and ½ inch up the sides of an 8×4×2-inch loaf pan; set aside. In a large bowl stir together flour, 1 cup sugar, baking powder, and salt. Make a well in the center of flour mixture; set aside.

2 | In a medium bowl combine milk, egg, oil, tangerine peel, 2 tablespoons tangerine juice, and poppy seeds. Add egg mixture all at once to flour mixture. Stir just until moistened (batter should be lumpy). Spoon batter into the prepared loaf pan, spreading evenly.

3 | Bake for 50 to 55 minutes or until a wooden toothpick inserted near the center comes out clean. Cool in pan on a wire rack for 10 minutes.

4 | Meanwhile, for glaze, in a small saucepan combine 2 tablespoons sugar, 2 tablespoons tangerine juice, and butter. Cook and stir over medium-low heat until butter is melted and sugar is dissolved.

5 | Remove bread from pan. Poke several holes in the top of the warm loaf with a long wooden skewer, making sure to poke down to the bottom of the loaf; slowly brush with glaze. Cool completely on wire rack. Wrap and store overnight before slicing.

*SUGAR SUBSTITUTE: Choose Splenda Sugar Blend for Baking. Follow package directions to use product amounts equivalent to 1 cup sugar and 2 tablespoons sugar.

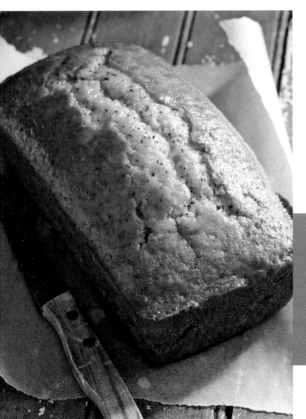

PER SERVING: 163 cal., 5 g total fat (1 g sat. fat), 14 mg chol., 151 mg sodium, 28 g carb. (1 g fiber, 15 g sugars), 3 g pro. Exchanges: 1 starch, 1 carb., 1 fat.

PER SERVING WITH SUBSTITUTE: Same as above, except 142 cal., 20 g carb. (8 g sugars). Exchanges: 0.5 carb.

Gluten-Free Zucchini Bread

Keep flours fresh longer by placing each in a freezer container or bag, then store in the freezer.

SERVINGS 16 (1 slice each)
CARB. PER SERVING 22 g or 19 g
PREP 20 minutes **STAND** 1 hour
BAKE 1 hour 5 minutes **COOL** 10 minutes

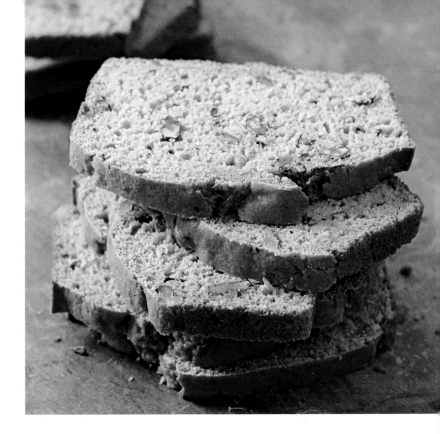

1	medium zucchini (8 ounces)
½	teaspoon salt
	Nonstick cooking spray
1½	cups gluten-free oat flour
1	cup gluten-free all-purpose flour
½	cup almond flour
½	cup sugar*
⅓	cup vanilla-flavor whey protein powder
2	teaspoons baking powder
1	teaspoon ground cinnamon
½	teaspoon ground ginger
¼	teaspoon ground cloves
6	ounces plain fat-free Greek yogurt
2	eggs
¾	cup unsweetened almond milk
½	cup chopped walnuts

PER SERVING: 167 cal., 6 g total fat (1 g sat. fat), 28 mg chol., 159 mg sodium, 22 g carb. (3 g fiber, 8 g sugars), 8 g pro. Exchanges: 1 starch, 0.5 carb., 1 lean meat, 0.5 fat.

PER SERVING WITH SUBSTITUTE: Same as above, except 157 cal., 19 g carb. (4 g sugars). Exchanges: 0 carb.

1 | Coarsely shred zucchini (you should have about 2 cups shredded zucchini). Place shredded zucchini in a sieve set over a bowl. Sprinkle the salt over zucchini; toss to combine. Let stand for 1 hour to drain. Place zucchini between three layers of 100-percent-cotton cheesecloth or two or three layers of paper towels; squeeze out excess liquid. Set aside.

2 | Preheat oven to 325°F. Coat a 9×5×3-inch loaf pan with cooking spray; set aside.

3 | In a large bowl whisk together gluten-free oat flour, gluten-free all-purpose flour, almond flour, sugar, whey protein powder, baking powder, cinnamon, ginger, and cloves. In another large bowl whisk together yogurt and shredded zucchini. Add eggs and almond milk; stir until combined. Add flour mixture to zucchini mixture; stir until well mixed. Stir in walnuts.

4 | Spoon batter into prepared pan. Bake for 65 to 75 minutes or until a wooden toothpick inserted in the center comes out with only a few moist crumbs attached.

5 | Cool in pan on a wire rack for 10 minutes. Run a thin metal spatula around the sides; turn out onto the wire rack. Cool completely before slicing.

*****SUGAR SUBSTITUTES:** Choose from Splenda Sugar Blend or C&H Light Sugar Blend. Follow package directions to use product amount equivalent to ½ cup sugar.

Peppered Pear Scones

Scones aren't just for breakfast. This savory variety pairs well with roasted or grilled chicken, pork, and lamb.

SERVINGS 16 (1 scone each)
CARB. PER SERVING 16 g or 14 g
PREP 25 minutes **BAKE** 10 minutes

- 1¾ cups flour
- ⅓ cup packed brown sugar*
- 2 teaspoons baking powder
- ½ teaspoon peppercorn melange or whole black peppercorns, cracked
- ¼ teaspoon baking soda
- ¼ teaspoon salt
- ⅓ cup unsalted butter
- 2 eggs
- ¼ cup grated Parmigiano-Reggiano cheese or Parmesan cheese (1 ounce)
- ¼ cup buttermilk or sour milk
- ½ cup chopped, peeled fresh pear, patted dry with paper towels

Peppercorn melange or whole black peppercorns, cracked (optional)

1 cup Pear Conserve (optional)

PER SERVING: 120 cal., 5 g total fat (3 g sat. fat), 35 mg chol., 136 mg sodium, 16 g carb. (1 g fiber, 5 g sugars), 3 g pro. Exchanges: 1 starch, 1 fat.

PER SERVING WITH SUBSTITUTE (SCONES ONLY): Same as above, except 113 cal., 134 mg sodium, 14 g carb. (3 g sugars).

1 | Preheat oven to 375°F. In a large bowl stir together flour, brown sugar, baking powder, ½ teaspoon cracked peppercorns, baking soda, and salt. Using a pastry blender, cut in butter until mixture resembles coarse crumbs. Make a well in the center of the flour mixture.

2 | In a small bowl lightly beat eggs; stir in cheese and buttermilk. Add the buttermilk mixture all at once to the flour mixture. Using a fork, stir just until moistened. Fold in pear.

3 | Turn out dough onto a floured surface. Knead dough by folding and gently pressing for 10 to 12 strokes or until dough is nearly smooth. Pat or lightly roll dough into an 8-inch square. Using a sharp large knife, cut into 16 squares. Place squares 1 inch apart on an ungreased baking sheet. If desired, sprinkle with additional cracked pepper.

4 | Bake for 10 to 12 minutes or until golden. Remove from baking sheet. Serve warm or at room temperature. If desired, serve with Pear Conserve.

PEAR CONSERVE: In a large saucepan combine 2½ cups chopped, peeled fresh pears; ½ cup water; and 3 tablespoons lemon juice. Bring to boiling; reduce heat. Simmer, covered, for 10 minutes. Stir in one 1.75-ounce package regular powdered fruit pectin. Bring to a full rolling boil, stirring constantly. Stir in 1¾ cups granulated sugar* and ½ cup golden raisins. Return to a full rolling boil. Boil hard for 1 minute, stirring constantly. Remove from heat; stir in ¼ teaspoon ground mace or cinnamon, and, if desired, ⅓ cup chopped toasted pecans or walnuts. Cool slightly. Ladle into an airtight storage container. Cover and seal. Store in the refrigerator for up to 3 days.

*SUGAR SUBSTITUTES: Choose Splenda Brown Sugar Blend for Baking for the scones. Follow package directions to use product amount equivalent to ⅓ cup brown sugar. If preparing, choose Splenda Sugar Blend for Baking for the conserve. Follow package directions to use product amount equivalent to 1¾ cups granulated sugar.

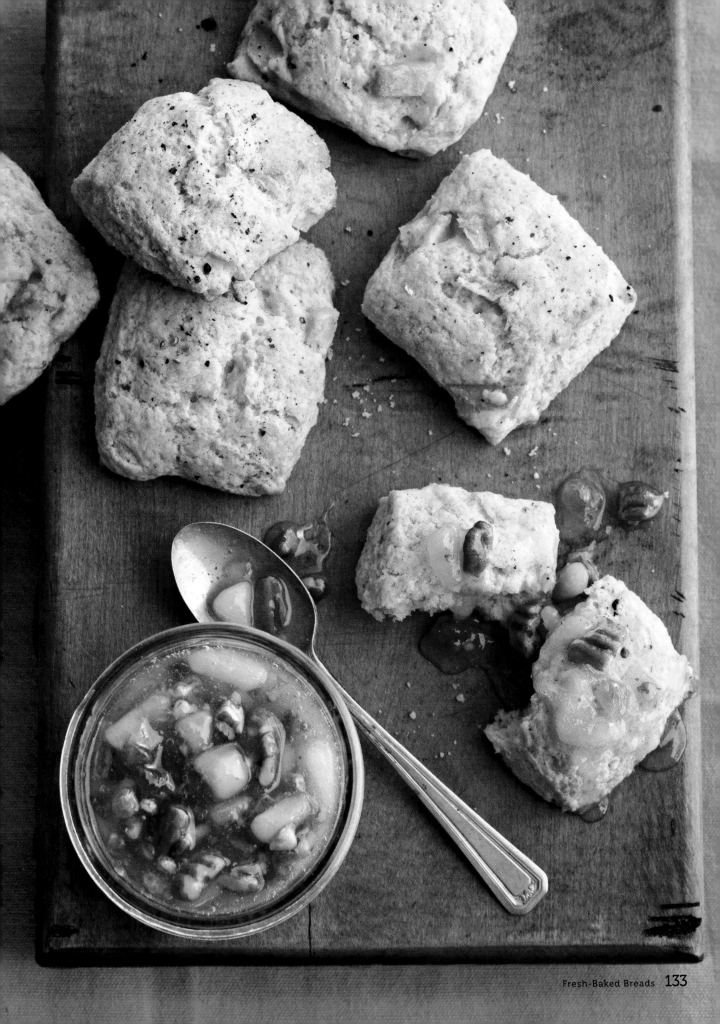

Mini Cranberry-Chocolate Scones

Rich and wonderful, each bite-size morsel is bursting with chocolaty good flavor.

SERVINGS 64 (1 mini scone each)
CARB. PER SERVING 7 g
PREP 20 minutes **BAKE** 8 minutes

2½ cups flour

2 tablespoons sugar*

1 tablespoon baking powder

¼ teaspoon salt

⅓ cup butter

2 eggs, lightly beaten

¾ cup whipping cream

¼ cup snipped dried cranberries

¼ cup miniature semisweet chocolate pieces

½ teaspoon finely shredded orange peel (optional)

1 tablespoon milk

1 recipe Orange Drizzle

1 Preheat oven to 400°F. In a large bowl stir together flour, sugar, baking powder, and salt. Using a pastry blender, cut in butter until mixture resembles coarse crumbs. Make a well in the center of the flour mixture; set aside.

2 In a medium bowl combine eggs, cream, dried cranberries, chocolate pieces, and, if desired, orange peel. Add egg mixture all at once to flour mixture. Using a fork, stir just until moistened.

3 Turn out dough onto a lightly floured surface. Knead dough by folding and gently pressing it for 10 to 12 strokes or until dough is nearly smooth. Pat or lightly roll dough into an 8-inch square. Using a sharp large knife, cut into 1-inch squares. Place squares 1 inch apart on an ungreased baking sheet. Brush with milk.

4 Bake for 8 to 10 minutes or until golden. Cool slightly on baking sheet. Drizzle with Orange Drizzle. Serve warm or at room temperature.

ORANGE DRIZZLE: In a small bowl combine 1 cup powdered sugar, 1 tablespoon orange juice, and ¼ teaspoon vanilla. Stir in additional orange juice, 1 teaspoon at a time, to reach a drizzling consistency.

*SUGAR SUBSTITUTES: Choose from Splenda Sugar Blend for Baking or C&H Light Blend. Follow package directions to use product amount equivalent to 2 tablespoons sugar.

TO STORE: Place iced scones in a single layer in an airtight container; cover. Store at room temperature for up to 2 days.

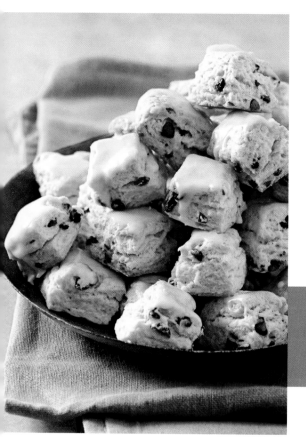

PER SERVING: 54 cal., 2 g total fat (1 g sat. fat), 12 mg chol., 38 mg sodium, 7 g carb. (0 g fiber, 3 g sugars), 1 g pro. Exchanges: 0.5 carb., 0.5 fat.

PER SERVING WITH SUBSTITUTE: Same as above.

Cheddar Biscuits

Choose these rich and cheesy biscuits to serve alongside juicy roasted beef or fill as breakfast sandwiches like on *page 15*.

SERVINGS 8 (1 biscuit each)
CARB. PER SERVING 22 g
PREP 20 minutes **BAKE** 14 minutes

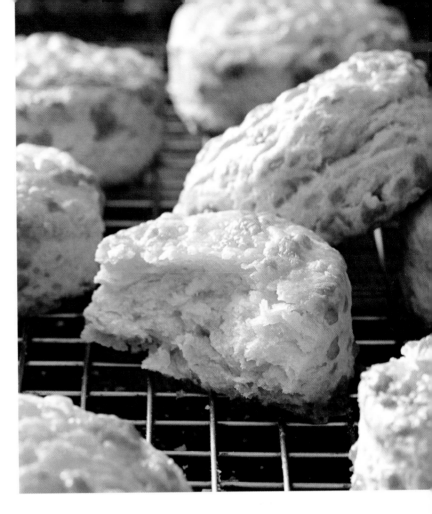

- 1³⁄₄ cups flour
- 2 teaspoons baking powder
- ¼ teaspoon salt
- 2 tablespoons cold butter, cut up
- 2 tablespoons plain fat-free Greek yogurt
- 1 tablespoon canola oil
- ¼ cup reduced-fat shredded cheddar cheese (1 ounce)
- ²⁄₃ cup fat-free milk

PER SERVING: 159 cal., 6 g total fat (3 g sat. fat), 11 mg chol., 253 mg sodium, 22 g carb. (1 g fiber, 1 g sugars), 5 g pro. Exchanges: 1.5 starch, 1 fat.

1 | Preheat oven to 425°F. In a large bowl stir together flour, baking powder, and salt. Using a pastry blender, cut in butter, yogurt, and oil until mixture resembles coarse crumbs. Stir in cheese. Make a well in the center of the flour mixture. Add milk all at once. Using a fork, stir just until moistened.

2 | Turn out dough onto a lightly floured surface. Knead dough by folding and gently pressing dough just until it holds together. Pat dough into an 8¹⁄₂×4¹⁄₂-inch rectangle. Cut dough lengthwise in half. Cut each half crosswise into four biscuits. Place biscuits 1 inch apart on an ungreased baking sheet.

3 | Bake about 14 minutes or until golden brown. Serve warm.

TO STORE: Place any remaining biscuits in an airtight container. Cover and store in the refrigerator for up to 2 days or freeze for up to 2 months.

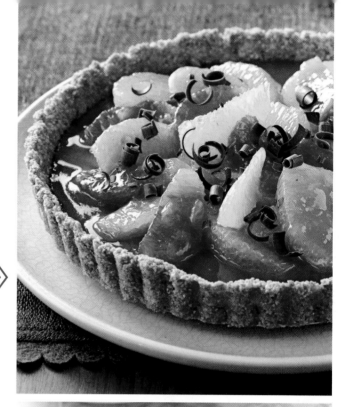

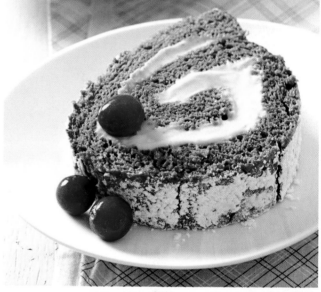

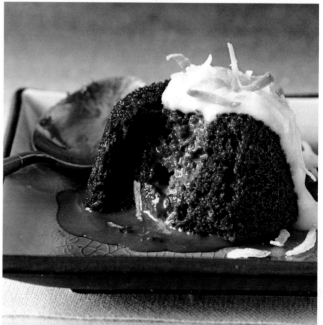

festive
endings

Holiday meals, no matter how sophisticated or casual, typically

end with a sweet finale. Having special dietary needs to

fulfill doesn't mean you can't indulge. A few tweaks here and

there have given these treats full flavor on a "light" calorie,

carbohydrate, and fat budget.

Sugar and Spice Popcorn Clusters

For chocolaty clusters without the heat, omit the chili powder and crushed red pepper.

SERVINGS 20 (1 cluster each)
CARB. PER SERVING 13 g
PREP 20 minutes **STAND** 3 hours

1½ cups dark chocolate pieces

2 teaspoons shortening

2 teaspoons chili powder

1 teaspoon ground cinnamon

¼ teaspoon crushed red pepper

6 cups popped 94% fat-free microwave popcorn (most of 1 bag) or air-popped popcorn

½ ounce white baking chocolate, melted

Chili powder and/or crushed red pepper (optional)

1 In a large microwave-safe bowl combine dark chocolate pieces and shortening. Microwave, uncovered, on 100 percent power (high) for 1½ to 2 minutes or until chocolate melts, stirring every 30 seconds.

2 In a small bowl combine the 2 teaspoons chili powder, the cinnamon, and the ¼ teaspoon crushed red pepper. Stir spice mixture into the melted chocolate mixture.

3 Slightly crush the popped popcorn;* stir crushed popcorn into the spiced chocolate mixture. Stir until the popcorn is evenly coated. Using two spoons, spoon popcorn mixture into 20 mounds onto waxed paper. Drizzle tops of the mounds with melted white baking chocolate. If desired, sprinkle with additional chili powder and/or crushed red pepper.

4 Let stand for 3 to 4 hours or until completely set before serving.

*TEST KITCHEN TIP: To crush the popcorn, place popped popcorn in a resealable plastic bag; seal bag. Using a rolling pin, lightly pound and roll popcorn until slightly crushed.

PER SERVING: 99 cal., 6 g total fat (4 g sat. fat), 0 mg chol., 21 mg sodium, 13 g carb. (2 g fiber, 10 g sugars), 1 g pro. Exchanges: 1 starch, 1 fat.

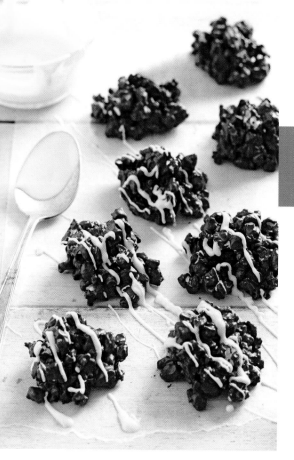

Peanut Cluster Butterscotch Bites

A classic peanutty candy mixture is nestled in flaky phyllo pastry cups to create mini tarts that are truly divine.

SERVINGS 45 (1 tart each)
CARB. PER SERVING 8 g
PREP 30 minutes STAND 15 minutes

- 1¼ cups semisweet chocolate pieces
- ½ cup butterscotch-flavor pieces
- ⅓ cup fat-free half-and-half
- 1 cup unsalted peanuts
- 45 baked miniature frozen phyllo shells
- ¼ cup unsalted peanuts, finely chopped
- Flaked sea salt (optional)

PER SERVING: 85 cal., 5 g total fat (2 g sat. fat), 0 mg chol., 14 mg sodium, 8 g carb. (1 g fiber, 4 g sugars), 2 g pro. Exchanges: 0.5 starch, 1 fat.

1 | In a small saucepan heat chocolate pieces and butterscotch-flavor pieces over low heat until melted and smooth, stirring frequently. Stir in half-and-half until smooth. Stir in 1 cup peanuts.

2 | Immediately spoon peanut mixture evenly into phyllo shells, using about 2 teaspoons per shell. Before mixture is set, sprinkle tops with finely chopped peanuts and, if desired, flaked sea salt. Let stand at room temperature about 15 minutes or until chocolate mixture is set.

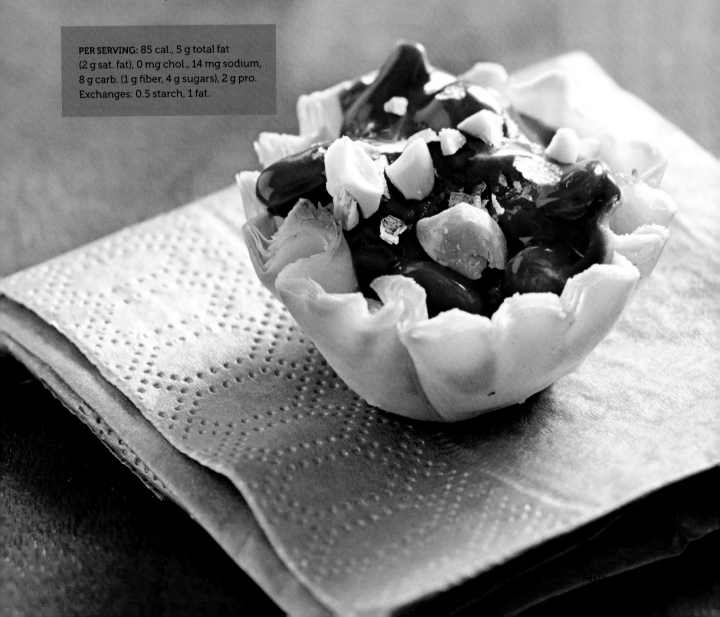

QUICK TIP
Carefully remove the sides of the tart pan before cutting the tart. Use a sharp knife to cut through the layers and wipe the knife clean between cuts.

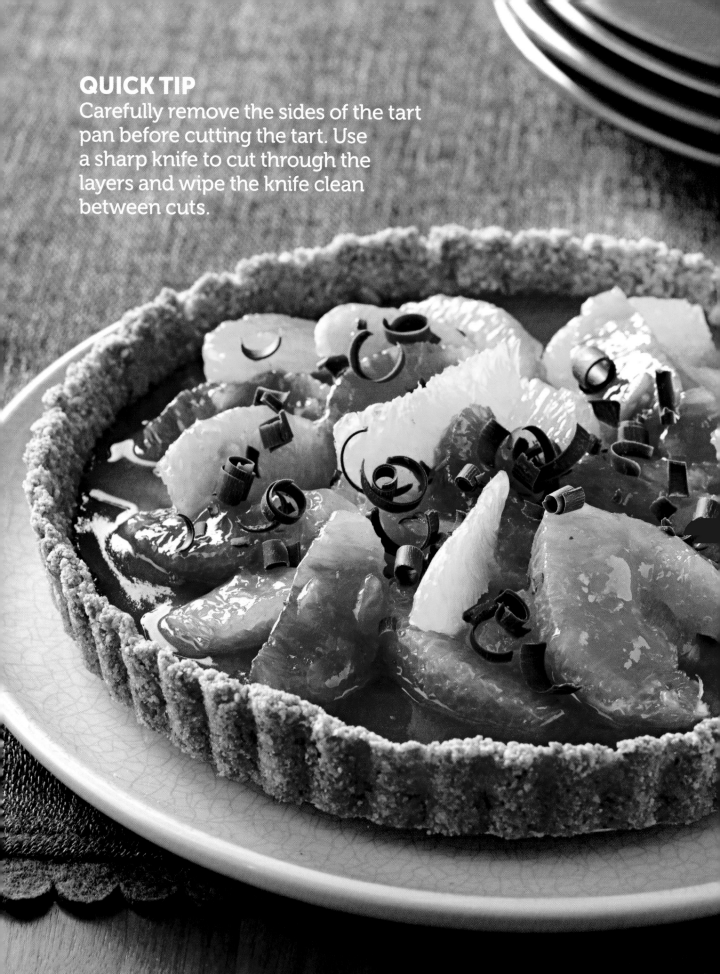

Decadent Orange-Chocolate Tart

Be as artistic as you like when arranging the orange slices on top of the creamy chocolate layer. Top the tart just before serving or the oranges will juice out too much.

SERVINGS 12 (1 slice each)
CARB. PER SERVING 27 g or 23 g
PREP 15 minutes **BAKE** 10 minutes
COOK 15 minutes **CHILL** overnight

1¼ cups finely crushed reduced-fat graham cracker squares (about 18)

3 tablespoons sugar*

½ teaspoon ground ginger

3 tablespoons butter, melted

1 egg white

6 tablespoons sugar*

¼ cup unsweetened cocoa powder

⅛ teaspoon salt

¾ cup fat-free half-and-half

4 egg yolks, lightly beaten

1 tablespoon butter

½ teaspoon vanilla

4 medium blood oranges, cara cara oranges, and/or navel oranges, peeled and sectioned

6 kumquats, thinly sliced crosswise (optional)

2 tablespoons sugar-free orange marmalade, melted

1 ounce dark chocolate curls

PER SERVING: 182 cal., 8 g total fat (4 g sat. fat), 72 mg chol., 131 mg sodium, 27 g carb. (2 g fiber, 19 g sugars), 3 g pro. Exchanges: 0.5 fruit, 0.5 starch, 1 carb., 1.5 fat.

PER SERVING WITH SUBSTITUTE: Same as above, except 168 cal., 23 g carb. (14 g sugars). Exchanges: 0.5 carb.

1 Preheat oven to 350°F. For crust, in a medium bowl combine graham cracker crumbs, the 3 tablespoons sugar, and ginger. In a small bowl beat butter and egg white together with a fork. Drizzle over graham cracker mixture; toss gently to mix. Press crumb mixture evenly onto bottom and up the sides of an 8-inch tart pan with removable bottom. Bake for 10 minutes. Remove from oven and cool in pan on a wire rack.

2 For filling, in a medium heavy saucepan combine the 6 tablespoons sugar, cocoa powder, and salt. Stir in half-and-half. Cook and stir over medium heat until mixture just comes to a simmer. Remove from heat. Gradually stir ½ cup of the half-and-half mixture into egg yolks. Add egg mixture to half-and-half mixture in saucepan. Bring to a gentle boil, stirring constantly. Remove from heat. Stir in the 1 tablespoon butter and the vanilla. Pour filling into the cooled crust. Cover surface of filling with plastic wrap. Refrigerate overnight.

3 Just before serving, arrange orange sections and kumquat slices (if using) in concentric circles on top of chocolate filling in tart pan, alternating the different colors of oranges randomly. Brush orange sections with the melted orange marmalade. Carefully remove sides of tart pan. Place tart on a serving platter. Garnish with chocolate curls. Cut into 12 slices.

*SUGAR SUBSTITUTE: Choose Splenda Sugar Blend for Baking. Follow package directions to use product amounts equivalent to 3 tablespoons and 6 tablespoons sugar.

Ginger-Pineapple Cheesecakes

A whole gingersnap cookie serves as the crust in each individual cheesecake. Be sure the cookies are not more than 2 inches across or you will need to cut them to fit.

SERVINGS 12 (1 cheesecake each)
CARB. PER SERVING 15 g or 14 g
PREP 25 minutes **BAKE** 15 minutes
COOL 20 minutes **CHILL** 1 hour

Nonstick cooking spray

15 2-inch gingersnap cookies

1 8-ounce package reduced-fat cream cheese (Neufchâtel)

1 6-ounce carton pineapple fat-free Greek yogurt

2 tablespoons sugar*

1 tablespoon flour

1 teaspoon vanilla

¾ teaspoon ground ginger

6 tablespoons refrigerated or frozen egg product, thawed

1 8-ounce can crushed pineapple (juice pack), very well drained

2 tablespoons finely chopped crystallized ginger

1 | Preheat oven to 350°F. Line twelve 2½-inch muffin cups with paper bake cups. Coat paper bake cups with cooking spray. Press one gingersnap into the bottom of each bake cup. Finely crush the remaining three gingersnap cookies; set aside.

2 | In a medium bowl beat cream cheese with an electric mixer on medium speed until smooth. Add yogurt, sugar, flour, vanilla, and ground ginger, beating until combined. Stir in egg; stir in drained pineapple and 1 tablespoon of the crystallized ginger. Divide batter evenly among the prepared bake cups. Sprinkle the remaining 1 tablespoon crystallized ginger and the reserved crushed gingersnaps over batter in cups.

3 | Bake about 15 minutes or until cheesecakes appear set. Cool in muffin cups on a wire rack for 20 minutes. Remove cheesecakes from muffin cups; cool completely on a wire rack. Cover and chill for 1 to 4 hours. To serve, remove from paper bake cups.

*SUGAR SUBSTITUTES: Choose from Splenda Granular, Truvia Spoonable, or Sweet'N Low bulk or packets. Follow package directions to use product amount equivalent to 2 tablespoons sugar.

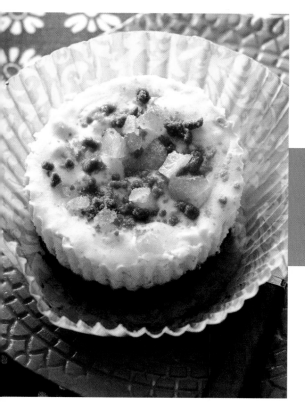

PER SERVING: 124 cal., 5 g total fat (2 g sat. fat), 14 mg chol., 143 mg sodium, 15 g carb. (0 g fiber, 11 g sugars), 4 g pro. Exchanges: 1 starch, 1 fat.

PER SERVING WITH SUBSTITUTE: Same as above, except 117 cal., 14 g carb. (9 g sugars).

Chocolate Meringues with Chocolate Topper

Here's a recipe designed just for two. Double or triple the recipe to serve more.

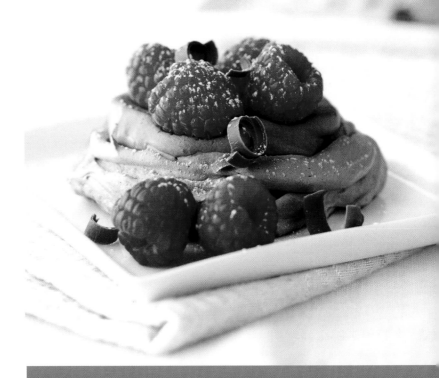

SERVINGS 2 (1 meringue shell, 1/4 cup raspberries, and about 3 tablespoons chocolate topper each)
CARB. PER SERVING 30 g
PREP 25 minutes **STAND** 30 minutes
BAKE 1 hour 30 minutes **STAND** 2 hours

- 1 egg white
- 1/8 teaspoon cream of tartar
- 1/8 teaspoon vanilla
- 1/3 cup powdered sugar
- 2 teaspoons unsweetened cocoa powder
- 1/3 cup frozen light whipped dessert topping, thawed
- 1 1/2 teaspoons unsweetened cocoa powder
- 1/2 cup fresh raspberries
- Powdered sugar (optional)
- Chocolate curls (optional)

PER SERVING: 142 cal., 2 g total fat (1 g sat. fat), 0 mg chol., 28 mg sodium, 30 g carb. (3 g fiber, 22 g sugars), 3 g pro. Exchanges: 2 carb.

1 For meringues, let egg white stand at room temperature for 30 minutes. Line a baking sheet with parchment paper or foil. Draw two 3-inch circles on the paper or foil; set aside.

2 Preheat oven to 200°F. In a medium bowl combine egg white, cream of tartar, and vanilla. Sift together the 1/3 cup powdered sugar and the 2 teaspoons cocoa powder; set aside. Beat egg white mixture with an electric mixer on medium speed until soft peaks form (tips curl). Add powdered sugar mixture, 1 tablespoon at a time, beating on high speed until stiff peaks form (tips stand straight).

3 Spoon or pipe meringue over circles on paper. Bake for 1 1/2 hours. Turn off oven; let meringues dry in oven with door closed for 2 hours. Lift meringues off paper; transfer to a wire rack.

4 For chocolate topper, place whipped topping in a small bowl. Fold in the 1 1/2 teaspoons cocoa powder. Chill until ready to serve.

5 To serve, spread the chocolate topper evenly onto meringues. Top with raspberries. If desired, dust lightly with additional powdered sugar and garnish with chocolate curls.

Chai Carrot Cake with Walnuts

Just before serving, stack the chilled frosted cake layers and garnish the top with the walnuts and, if desired, carrot shreds and ground nutmeg.

SERVINGS 16 (1 piece each)
CARB. PER SERVING 33 g or 26 g
PREP 45 minutes BAKE 20 minutes
CHILL 1 hour

- 2 spiced chai tea bags
- 1½ cups all-purpose flour
- ⅓ cup whole wheat pastry flour or whole wheat flour
- 3 tablespoons flaxseed meal
- 2 teaspoons baking powder
- ½ teaspoon baking soda
- ¼ teaspoon salt
- 2½ cups finely shredded carrots (about 5 medium)
- 1 cup refrigerated or frozen egg product, thawed, or 4 eggs, lightly beaten
- ½ cup granulated sugar*
- ½ cup packed brown sugar*
- ½ cup unsweetened applesauce
- ⅓ cup canola oil
- 1 recipe Spicy Cream Cheese Frosting**
- ⅓ cup coarsely chopped walnuts, toasted

PER SERVING: 227 cal., 9 g total fat (2 g sat. fat), 7 mg chol., 209 mg sodium, 33 g carb. (2 g fiber, 19 g sugars), 5 g pro. Exchanges: 1 starch, 1 carb., 1.5 fat.

PER SERVING WITH SUBSTITUTE: Same as above, except 206 cal., 207 sodium, 26 g carb. (12 g sugars).

1 Preheat oven to 350°F. Grease two 8×1½- or 9×1½-inch round cake pans; line bottom of pans with waxed paper. Grease and lightly flour the waxed paper and the sides of the pans. Set aside. Cut tea bags open and pour tea mixture into a spice grinder or mortar and pestle; grind to a fine powder.

2 In a large bowl combine ground tea mixture, the flours, flaxseed meal, baking powder, baking soda, and salt; set aside. In another large bowl combine finely shredded carrots, egg, granulated sugar, brown sugar, applesauce, and oil. Add egg mixture all at once to flour mixture. Stir until combined. Divide batter evenly between prepared pans; spread evenly.

3 Bake for 25 to 30 minutes for 8-inch pans, 20 to 25 minutes for 9-inch pans, or until a toothpick inserted near centers comes out clean. Cool cakes in pans on wire racks for 10 minutes. Invert cakes onto racks. Cool completely.

4 Prepare Spicy Cream Cheese Frosting.** Place a cooled cake layer on a serving plate. Top with half of the frosting. Place a second cake layer on another plate; spread with remaining frosting. Chill layers for 1 hour. Place one layer on top of layer on the serving plate. Sprinkle top with walnuts.

SPICY CREAM CHEESE FROSTING: In a small saucepan sprinkle 1 teaspoon unflavored gelatin over 2 tablespoons cold water. Let stand for 5 minutes. Stir over medium-low heat until gelatin is dissolved. Remove from heat; stir in ¼ cup honey. Transfer to a medium bowl. Beat with a handheld electric mixer on high speed for 5 to 7 minutes or until mixture lightens and expands to about 1¼ cups. In another medium bowl beat 4 ounces softened reduced-fat cream cheese (Neufchâtel) with the mixer on medium speed for 30 seconds. Gradually beat in ½ cup light sour cream until smooth. Beat in ½ teaspoon vanilla, ⅛ teaspoon ground cardamom, ⅛ teaspoon ground nutmeg, and ⅛ teaspoon ground cinnamon. Fold in about one-fourth of the honey mixture. Fold in remaining honey mixture.

*SUGAR SUBSTITUTES: Choose Splenda Blend for Baking to substitute for the granulated sugar. Choose Splenda Brown Sugar Blend for Baking to substitute for the brown sugar. Follow package directions to use product amounts equivalent to ½ cup each granulated and brown sugars.

**TEST KITCHEN TIP: Don't prepare the frosting until you are ready to frost the cake.

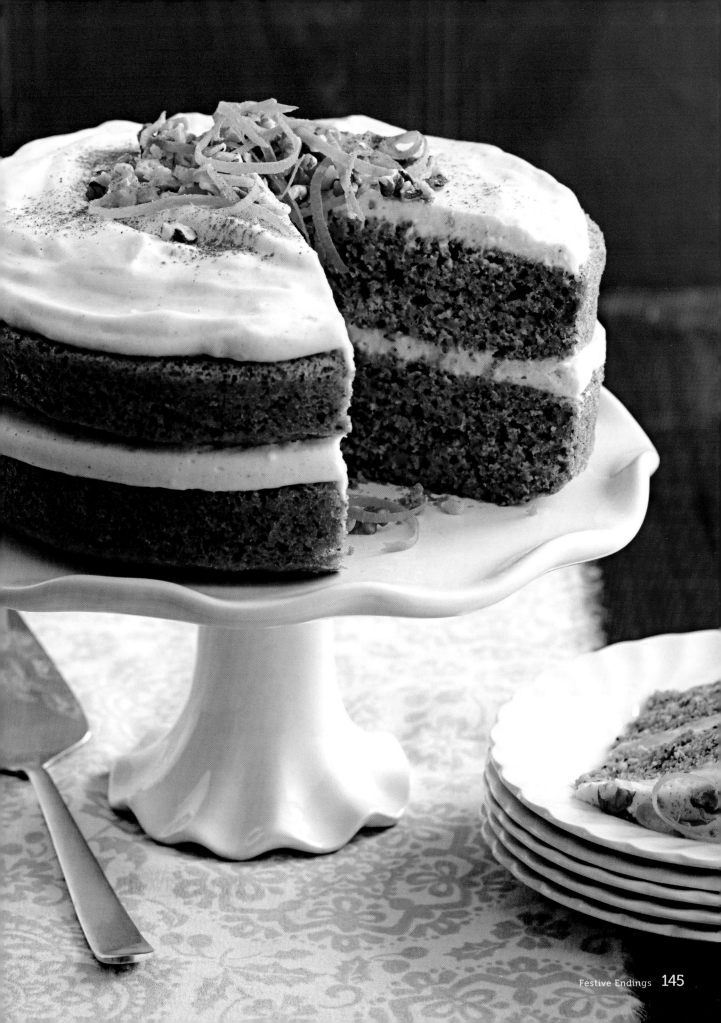

Cran-Raspberry Shortcakes

Shortcake, a summertime favorite, gets a wintertime makeover. Fresh cranberries and frozen raspberries star in the saucy topping.

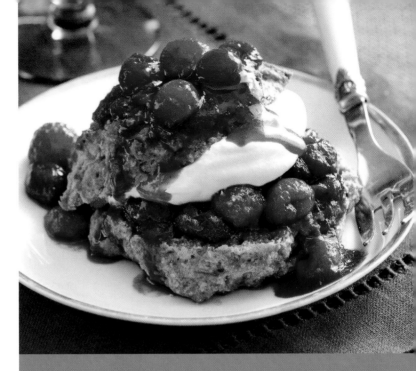

SERVINGS 10 (1 biscuit, 3 tablespoons sauce, and 1 tablespoon whipped topping each)
CARB. PER SERVING 31 g or 27 g
PREP 25 minutes **BAKE** 12 minutes
COOK 15 minutes

¼ teaspoon canola oil
1 cup all-purpose flour
½ cup whole wheat flour
¼ cup sugar*
2 teaspoons baking powder
1¼ teaspoons ground cinnamon
¼ teaspoon salt
¼ cup butter
1 egg
1 6-ounce carton plain fat-free Greek yogurt
¼ cup fat-free milk
¾ cup water
1½ cups fresh or frozen cranberries
½ cup 100% juice cranberry blend
2 tablespoons sugar*
2 tablespoons balsamic vinegar
2 cups frozen unsweetened raspberries
10 tablespoons frozen light whipped dessert topping, thawed

PER SERVING: 196 cal., 6 g total fat (4 g sat. fat), 31 mg chol., 216 mg sodium, 31 g carb. (3 g fiber, 13 g sugars), 5 g pro. Exchanges: 1 fruit, 1 starch, 1 fat.

PER SERVING WITH SUBSTITUTE: Same as above, except 184 cal., 27 g carb. (9 g sugars).

1 Preheat oven to 400°F. Grease a large baking sheet with the canola oil. In a large bowl combine flours, the ¼ cup sugar, the baking powder, cinnamon, and salt. Using a pastry blender, cut in butter until mixture resembles coarse crumbs. In a small bowl whisk together egg, yogurt, and milk. Add yogurt mixture to flour mixture; stir just until moistened (if needed, toss in 2 to 4 tablespoons water). Drop dough into 10 mounds on the prepared baking sheet. Bake for 12 to 15 minutes or until golden brown and a wooden toothpick inserted near centers comes out clean.

2 Meanwhile, for sauce, in a medium saucepan combine the ¾ cup water, cranberries, juice blend, sugar, and vinegar. Bring to boiling over medium heat; reduce heat. Simmer, uncovered, about 15 minutes or until thickened, stirring frequently. Remove from heat; stir in frozen raspberries. Cool slightly.

3 Split shortcakes; arrange on individual serving plates. Spoon half of the sauce over the shortcake bottoms. Add a spoonful of whipped topping and add the shortcake tops. Top with remaining sauce.

*SUGAR SUBSTITUTES: Choose from Splenda Sugar Blend, C&H Light Sugar Blend, or Truvia Baking Blend. Follow package directions to use product amounts equivalent to ¼ cup sugar for the shortcakes and 2 tablespoons sugar for the sauce.

Clementine-Clove Snowballs

The cake mixture may be sticky, so dampening your hands to shape it into balls may be helpful.

SERVINGS 24 (1 snowball each)
CARB. PER SERVING 22 g
PREP 1 hour BAKE according to package
FREEZE 1 hour CHILL 1 hour

- 1 16-ounce package angel food cake mix

  Orange juice

- ½ teaspoon ground cloves

- 1 8-ounce package reduced-fat cream cheese (Neufchâtel), softened

- 2 6-ounce cartons orange creme-flavor sugar-free, fat-free yogurt

- 1 cup finely chopped, peeled clementines (4 to 5)

- 1½ cups frozen light whipped dessert topping, thawed

- ½ teaspoon unsweetened cocoa powder

  Halved clementine slices (optional)

1 Prepare cake mix according to package directions, except substitute orange juice for the water called for on the package (this is usually 1¼ cups) and add the ground cloves to the dry mix. Use any suggested pan size and bake according to package directions. Cool cake in pan on a wire rack; remove cake from pan. Line trays with waxed paper; set aside.

2 In a very large bowl beat cream cheese with an electric mixer on medium speed until smooth. Add one carton of the yogurt, beating until smooth. Stir in finely chopped clementines. Crumble cake into the cream cheese mixture. Beat with the electric mixer until combined. Drop cake mixture into 24 mounds on prepared trays or sheets, using about 3 tablespoons (No. 20 scoop) cake mixture for each mound. Roll mounds into balls (mixture will be sticky). Freeze about 1 hour or until balls are firm.*

3 In a medium bowl fold together the remaining yogurt and the dessert topping. Working with one cake ball at a time, insert a fork or wooden skewer carefully into each ball. Spread a thin layer of the topping mixture over each ball or dip each ball into topping, leaving the base of each ball unfrosted. Use a table knife or small metal spatula to gently push the coated ball off the fork and back onto the tray or sheet. If necessary, use the knife or spatula to spread the topping over area where fork was. Dust balls with cocoa powder. Chill for 1 to 24 hours before serving.

4 To serve, place snowballs on a cake plate and, if desired, garnish with halved clementine slices.

*MAKE-AHEAD DIRECTIONS: If desired, prepare as directed in Steps 1 and 2, except omit freezing the balls until firm and place balls in airtight containers. Store in the refrigerator for up to 3 days or freeze for up to 1 month. If frozen, let stand at room temperature for 30 minutes before continuing as directed in Steps 3 and 4.

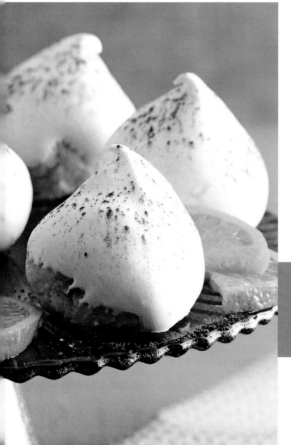

PER SERVING: 124 cal., 3 g total fat (2 g sat. fat), 7 mg chol., 199 mg sodium, 22 g carb. (0 g fiber, 15 g sugars), 3 g pro. Exchanges: 0.5 fruit, 1 starch, 0.5 fat.

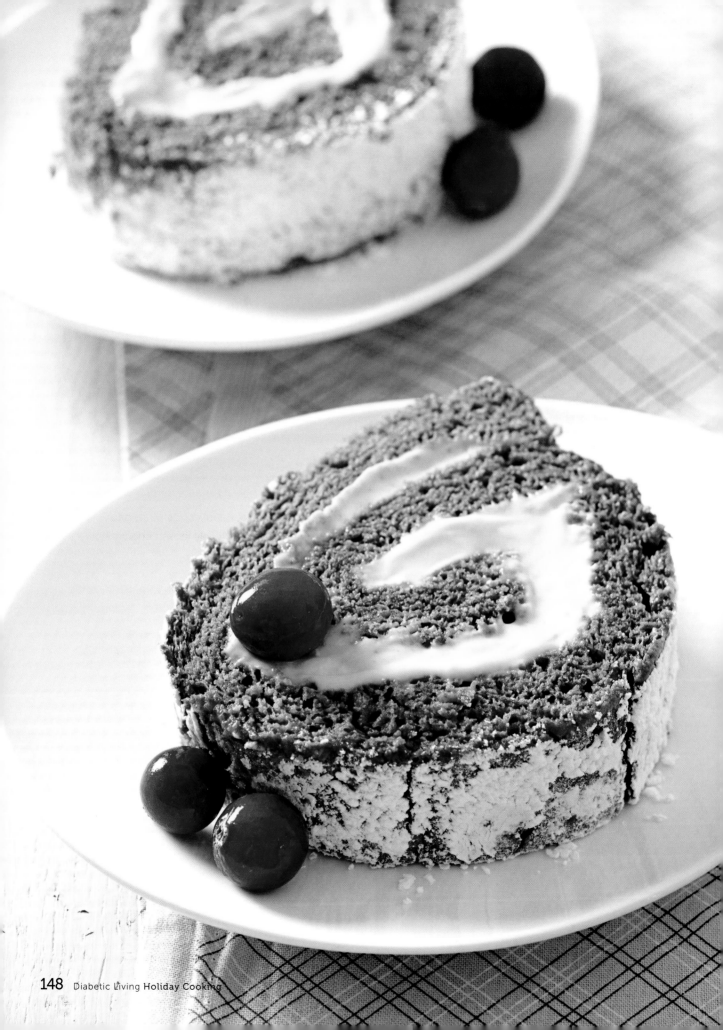

Spice Cake Roll with Cream Cheese Filling

Cut the cake with a long serrated knife, using a gentle back-and-forth motion. The filling will ooze out if you have a heavy hand.

SERVINGS 12 (1 slice each)
CARB. PER SERVING 27 g
PREP 35 minutes **BAKE** 12 minutes
STAND 40 minutes
COOK 5 minutes **CHILL** 4 hours

- 4 eggs
- 1/3 cup all-purpose flour
- 1/4 cup whole wheat pastry flour or whole wheat flour
- 1 1/2 teaspoons pumpkin pie spice
- 1 teaspoon baking powder
- 1/4 teaspoon salt
- 1/4 teaspoon ground cloves
- 1 teaspoon vanilla
- 1/2 cup full-flavor molasses
- 1/3 cup granulated sugar*
- Powdered sugar*
- 1/4 cup granulated sugar*
- 1 tablespoon cornstarch
- 1 cup fat-free milk
- 2 egg yolks, lightly beaten
- 6 ounces reduced-fat cream cheese (Neufchâtel), softened and cut up
- 1 teaspoon vanilla
- Powdered sugar* (optional)

PER SERVING: 180 cal., 6 g total fat (3 g sat. fat), 104 mg chol., 175 mg sodium, 27 g carb. (0 g fiber, 21 g sugars), 5 g pro. Exchanges: 0.5 starch, 1.5 carb., 0.5 medium-fat meat, 0.5 fat.

1 Separate eggs. Allow 4 egg whites and 4 egg yolks to stand at room temperature for 30 minutes. Meanwhile, grease a 15×10×1-inch baking pan. Line bottom of pan with waxed paper or parchment paper; grease paper. Set pan aside. In a medium bowl stir together flours, pumpkin pie spice, baking powder, salt, and cloves; set aside.

2 Preheat oven to 375°F. In a medium mixing bowl beat the 4 egg yolks and 1 teaspoon vanilla with an electric mixer on high speed about 5 minutes or until thick and lemon color. Beat in molasses just until combined.

3 Thoroughly wash beaters. In a large mixing bowl beat egg whites on medium speed until soft peaks form (tips curl). Gradually add the 1/3 cup sugar, beating until stiff peaks form (tips stand straight). Fold egg yolk mixture into beaten egg whites. Sprinkle flour mixture over egg mixture; fold in just until combined. Spread batter evenly in prepared baking pan.

4 Bake for 12 to 15 minutes or until cake springs back when lightly touched. Immediately loosen edges of cake from pan and turn cake out onto a clean kitchen towel generously sprinkled with powdered sugar. Remove waxed paper. Roll towel and cake into a spiral, starting from a short side of the cake. Cool on a wire rack.

5 For filling, in a heavy medium saucepan combine the 1/4 cup sugar and cornstarch. Gradually stir in milk. Cook and stir over medium heat until thickened and bubbly. Cook and stir for 1 minute more. Gradually stir half of the milk mixture into the 2 beaten egg yolks. Return yolk mixture to the pan. Bring just to a boil; reduce heat. Cook and stir for 2 minutes. Remove from heat. Add cream cheese and the 1 teaspoon vanilla. Let stand for 5 minutes. Whisk until smooth.

6 Place bowl with the filling in a larger bowl of ice water; let stand for 5 minutes, stirring occasionally. Cover surface with plastic wrap. Chill 4 hours or until cold; do not stir.

7 To assemble cake roll, unroll cake; remove towel. Spread cake with filling to within 1 inch of the edges. Roll up cake; trim ends. Cover and chill for up to 6 hours. If desired, before serving, sift powdered sugar over cake roll.

*SUGAR SUBSTITUTES: We do not recommend using sugar substitutes for this recipe.

Crackled Sugar Cookies

A low oven temperature and longer baking provide the perfect environment for the balls to melt, crackle, and dry into crispy cookies.

SERVINGS 48 (1 cookie each)
CARB. PER SERVING 12 g or 8 g
PREP 35 minutes **BAKE** 12 minutes per batch **STAND** 2 minutes

½   cup butter, softened
½   cup shortening
2   cups sugar*
1   teaspoon baking soda
1   teaspoon cream of tartar
⅛   teaspoon salt
3   egg yolks
½   teaspoon vanilla
1¾   cups flour

PER SERVING: 88 cal., 4 g total fat (2 g sat. fat), 17 mg chol., 50 mg sodium, 12 g carb. (0 g fiber, 8 g sugars), 1 g pro. Exchanges: 1 carb., 1 fat.

PER SERVING WITH SUBSTITUTE: Same as above, except 66 cal., 8 g carb. (4 g sugars). Exchanges: 0.5 carb.

1 | Preheat oven to 300°F. In a large mixing bowl beat butter and shortening with an electric mixer on medium to high speed for 30 seconds. Add sugar, baking soda, cream of tartar, and salt. Beat mixture until combined, scraping sides of bowl occasionally. Beat in egg yolks and vanilla. Beat in as much of the flour as you can with the mixer. Stir in any remaining flour.

2 | Shape dough into 1-inch balls. Place balls 2 inches apart on ungreased cookie sheets.

3 | Bake for 12 to 14 minutes or until edges are set; do not let edges brown. Cool cookies for 2 minutes on cookie sheet. Transfer cookies to wire racks and let cool.

*SUGAR SUBSTITUTES: Choose from Splenda Sugar Blend for Baking or C&H Light Sugar and Stevia Blend. Follow package directions to use product amount equivalent to 2 cups sugar.

TO STORE: Layer cookies between waxed paper in an airtight container; cover. Store at room temperature for up to 2 days or label and freeze for up to 3 months.

QUICK TIP
For perfect rounds, use a small cookie scoop to portion the dough. Roll each portion into a ball with your hands.

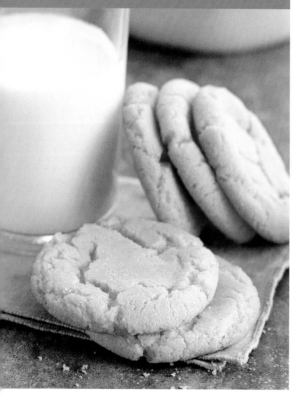

Raspberry Semifreddo with Pistachios

To plate each dessert individually, position a slice of semifreddo, add a spoonful of honeyed raspberries, and sprinkle with mint.

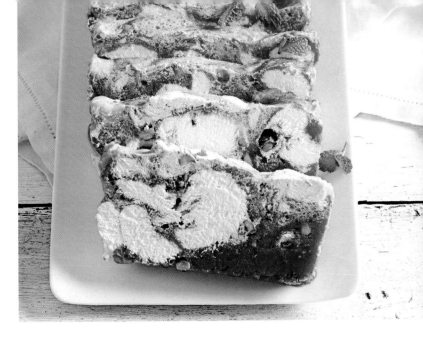

SERVINGS 12 (1 slice and 2 tablespoons raspberries each)
CARB. PER SERVING 22 g or 20 g
PREP 30 minutes **FREEZE** 6 hours
STAND 10 minutes

- 1 pound fresh or frozen red raspberries, thawed (3½ cups)
- ¼ cup sugar*
- 2 tablespoons lime juice
- Dash salt
- 3 eggs
- 1 8-ounce container frozen light whipped dessert topping, thawed
- ¼ teaspoon almond extract
- ½ cup chopped pistachio nuts
- 8 ounces fresh red raspberries (1¾ cups)
- 2 tablespoons honey
- Fresh mint leaves (optional)

PER SERVING: 147 cal., 6 g total fat (3 g sat. fat), 47 mg chol., 48 mg sodium, 22 g carb. (4 g fiber, 12 g sugars), 3 g pro. Exchanges: 0.5 fruit, 1 carb., 0.5 medium-fat meat, 0.5 fat.

PER SERVING WITH SUBSTITUTE: Same as above, except: 141 cal., 20 g carb. (10 g sugars). Exchanges: 0.5 carb.

1 | Line a 9×5×3-inch loaf pan with a double layer of plastic wrap, leaving a 2-inch overhang on all sides; set aside.

2 | In a food processor combine the 1 pound raspberries, 2 tablespoons of the sugar, the lime juice, and salt. Cover and process until pureed and smooth. Strain the puree through a fine-mesh sieve; discard seeds. Set puree aside.

3 | In a medium heatproof bowl combine eggs and the remaining 2 tablespoons sugar. Beat with an electric mixer on medium speed until combined. Place bowl over a saucepan filled with gently boiling water (the bowl should not touch the water). Cook, beating constantly on medium speed, until an instant-read thermometer inserted in center of the mixture registers 140°F and maintains that temperature for 3½ minutes (10 to 12 minutes total cooking time) or reaches 160°F. Remove pan from heat. Remove bowl from over the water; continue beating off the heat until cooled to room temperature (about 5 minutes).

4 | In a large bowl combine whipped topping and almond extract. Fold cooled egg mixture, the raspberry puree, and ½ cup pistachios into whipped topping mixture, leaving some swirls. Pour into prepared pan; smooth the top. Cover with plastic wrap; freeze for 6 to 24 hours or until firm.

5 | To serve, toss the 8 ounces fresh raspberries with honey. Remove semifreddo from freezer and let stand for 10 to 15 minutes to soften slightly. Remove semifreddo from pan by pulling up on the overhanging plastic wrap, then invert onto a cutting board and peel off plastic. Cut into 12 slices. If desired, garnish with fresh mint. Serve immediately with some of the honeyed raspberries.

***SUGAR SUBSTITUTE:** Choose Splenda Sugar Blend for Baking. Follow package directions to use product amount equivalent to ¼ cup sugar.

Walnut-Nutmeg Pumpkin Custards

A spoonful of this streusel-topped spiced custard is like eating pumpkin pie without the crust.

SERVINGS 8 (1 custard and 1 tablespoon topping each)
CARB. PER SERVING 31 g or 30 g
PREP 25 minutes BAKE 30 minutes COOL 30 minutes CHILL 2 hours

Nonstick cooking spray

1 cup evaporated fat-free milk

1 cup canned pumpkin

2 eggs, lightly beaten

2/3 cup pure maple syrup

1/2 cup refrigerated or frozen egg product, thawed

2 teaspoons vanilla

3/4 teaspoon ground nutmeg

1/4 teaspoon salt

1/4 teaspoon ground allspice

1/4 cup chopped walnuts

1/4 cup regular rolled oats

2 tablespoons packed brown sugar*

1 tablespoon butter, melted

1/2 cup frozen light whipped dessert topping, thawed

Freshly grated nutmeg (optional)

1 Preheat oven to 350°F. Coat eight 6-ounce ramekins with cooking spray. Place ramekins in two 2-quart square baking dishes.

2 In a medium bowl combine evaporated milk, pumpkin, eggs, maple syrup, egg product, and vanilla. In a small bowl sift together 1/2 teaspoon of the ground nutmeg, the salt, and allspice. Add spice mixture to the pumpkin mixture; beat with a wire whisk until well mixed.

3 In the small bowl that contained the spice mixture combine walnuts, oats, brown sugar, and the remaining 1/4 teaspoon ground nutmeg. Add melted butter; stir just until combined.

4 Divide pumpkin mixture evenly among the prepared ramekins. Place baking dishes on the oven rack. Pour enough boiling water into baking dishes to reach halfway up the sides of the ramekins. Bake for 15 minutes. Carefully top each with about 1 tablespoon of the nut mixture. Bake for 15 to 20 minutes more or until a knife inserted near centers comes out clean.

5 Remove ramekins from water; cool on a wire rack for 30 minutes. Cover and chill for 2 to 8 hours before serving. To serve, top with whipped dessert topping and, if desired, sprinkle with freshly grated nutmeg.

SUGAR SUBSTITUTE: Choose Splenda Brown Sugar Blend. Follow package directions to use product amount equivalent to 2 tablespoons brown sugar.

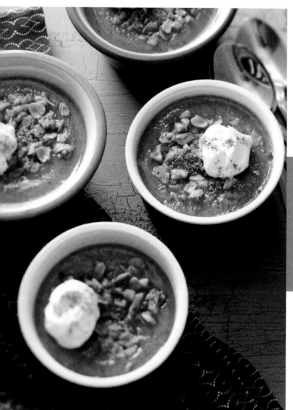

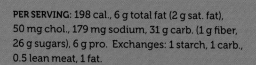

PER SERVING: 198 cal., 6 g total fat (2 g sat. fat), 50 mg chol., 179 mg sodium, 31 g carb. (1 g fiber, 26 g sugars), 6 g pro. Exchanges: 1 starch, 1 carb., 0.5 lean meat, 1 fat.

PER SERVING WITH SUBSTITUTE: Same as above, except 197 cal., 30 g carb.

Chocolate Ravioli

When baked, wonton wrappers make a crispy pastry that encases a cheesy chocolate filling. Add a drizzle of caramel for a spectacular presentation.

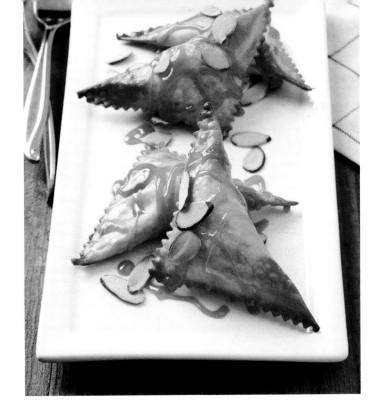

SERVINGS 10 (2 ravioli each)
CARB. PER SERVING 19 g or 17 g
PREP 20 minutes **BAKE** 12 minutes

Nonstick cooking spray

$\frac{1}{2}$ cup light cream cheese spread

2 tablespoons sugar*

2 ounces milk chocolate, finely chopped ($\frac{1}{3}$ cup)

20 wonton wrappers

1 egg

1 tablespoon water

2 tablespoons sugar-free caramel-flavor ice cream topping

1 tablespoon sliced almonds or chopped pecans, toasted

PER SERVING: 134 cal., 5 g total fat (3 g sat. fat), 29 mg chol., 165 mg sodium, 19 g carb. (0 g fiber, 7 g sugars), 3 g pro. Exchanges: 0.5 starch, 0.5 carb., 1 fat.

PER SERVING WITH SUBSTITUTE: Same as above, except 131 cal., 17 g carb. (5 g sugars).

1 | Preheat oven to 375°F. Line a large baking sheet with foil. Coat foil with cooking spray; set aside.

2 | For filling, in a small bowl stir together the cream cheese and sugar until smooth. Stir in the chopped chocolate.

3 | Lay a few wonton wrappers on a work surface. Cover remaining wonton wrappers while working to keep them from drying out. Spoon $1\frac{1}{2}$ teaspoons of the filling into the center of each wrapper. Lightly moisten the edges of each wrapper with water. Fold two opposite corners together, pressing edges to seal, to form triangles. If desired, use a fluted pastry wheel to trim edges of each triangle. In a small bowl whisk together the egg with the 1 tablespoon water. Brush egg mixture over each filled ravioli. Repeat with remaining wonton wrappers and filling.

4 | Place ravioli on prepared baking sheet. Bake for 12 to 14 minutes or until golden brown and crisp. Place ravioli on serving plates. Place caramel ice cream topping in a small resealable plastic bag; snip off a tiny corner of the bag. Pipe topping over the ravioli and sprinkle with almonds. Serve warm.

*SUGAR SUBSTITUTES: Choose from Splenda Sugar Blend for Baking or C&H Light Sugar and Stevia Blend. Follow package directions to use product amount equivalent to 2 tablespoons sugar.

Molten Chocolate Cakes with Coconut Cream

Make sure the table is set for dessert. Once the fluffy coconut mixture is spooned onto the warm cake, it begins to melt.

SERVINGS 6 (1 cake and 2 tablespoons coconut cream each)
CARB. PER SERVING 33 g or 25 g
PREP 30 minutes STAND 12 minutes BAKE 12 minutes

1/3 cup original-flavor refrigerated coconut milk beverage

3/4 teaspoon unflavored gelatin

3 tablespoons granulated sugar*

1/4 teaspoon clear vanilla

1/8 teaspoon coconut extract (optional)

1/2 cup flour

3 tablespoons unsweetened cocoa powder

1/4 teaspoon baking soda

1/8 teaspoon salt

2 egg whites

1/4 cup packed brown sugar*

2 tablespoons fat-free milk

2 tablespoons canola oil

1/2 teaspoon clear vanilla

1/4 cup dark chocolate pieces or chopped dark chocolate

3 tablespoons fat-free half-and-half

2 tablespoons shredded coconut, lightly toasted

1 For coconut cream, pour coconut milk into a medium stainless-steel bowl. Sprinkle gelatin over milk. Let stand for 5 minutes. Heat about 3 inches of water in a Dutch oven to simmering; place the bowl of milk mixture in Dutch oven. Heat over medium heat for 2 to 3 minutes or until gelatin is dissolved, stirring milk mixture frequently (the milk might look separated).

2 Carefully remove the bowl of milk mixture from the Dutch oven; place the bowl in a large bowl half-filled with ice. Add 1 tablespoon of the granulated sugar, the 1/4 teaspoon vanilla, and, if desired, coconut extract to milk mixture. Beat with an electric mixer on high speed for 3 to 8 minutes or until mixture is thickened and fluffy and stiff peaks form (tips stand straight). Set aside while making cakes.

3 For cakes, preheat oven to 350°F. Grease six 2½-inch muffin cups; set aside. In a medium bowl whisk together flour, cocoa powder, baking soda, and salt. In another medium bowl whisk together egg whites, brown sugar, the remaining 2 tablespoons granulated sugar, the fat-free milk, oil, and 1/2 teaspoon vanilla. Add all at once to the flour mixture. Whisk until well combined. Spoon evenly into prepared muffin cups.

4 Bake about 9 minutes or until puffed, edges are firm, and centers look like batter. Meanwhile, in a small microwave-safe bowl combine chocolate pieces and half-and-half. Microwave, uncovered, on 30 percent power (medium-low) for 1 to 1½ minutes or until chocolate is nearly melted, stirring once halfway through cooking. Let stand for 2 minutes. Stir until completely smooth.

5 Remove cakes from the oven. Use two forks to slightly open centers of the cakes. Spoon melted chocolate mixture evenly into centers of cakes (some of the melted chocolate will sit on top). Bake for 3 minutes more. Let stand in muffin cups on a wire rack for 5 minutes.

6 Use a thin knife to loosen cakes from edges of cups. If needed, use two spoons to carefully lift each cake out of cup. Invert cakes onto plates. Spoon coconut cream mixture on top; sprinkle with toasted coconut. Serve immediately.

QUICK TIP
To fill the cake centers, use two forks to gently pull apart the center of each cake, then use a tableware spoon to add the melted chocolate.

*SUGAR SUBSTITUTES: Choose from Splenda Sugar Blend for Baking or Equal Sugar Lite to substitute for the granulated sugar. Choose Splenda Brown Sugar Blend for Baking to substitute for the brown sugar. Follow package directions to use product amounts equivalent to 3 tablespoons granulated sugar and 1/4 cup brown sugar.

PER SERVING: 219 cal., 9 g total fat (3 g sat. fat), 0 mg chol., 143 mg sodium, 33 g carb. (2 g fiber, 22 g sugars), 5 g pro. Exchanges: 1 starch, 1 carb., 1.5 fat.

PER SERVING WITH SUBSTITUTE: Same as above, except 195 cal., 140 mg sodium, 25 g carb. (14 g sugars). Exchanges: 0.5 carb.

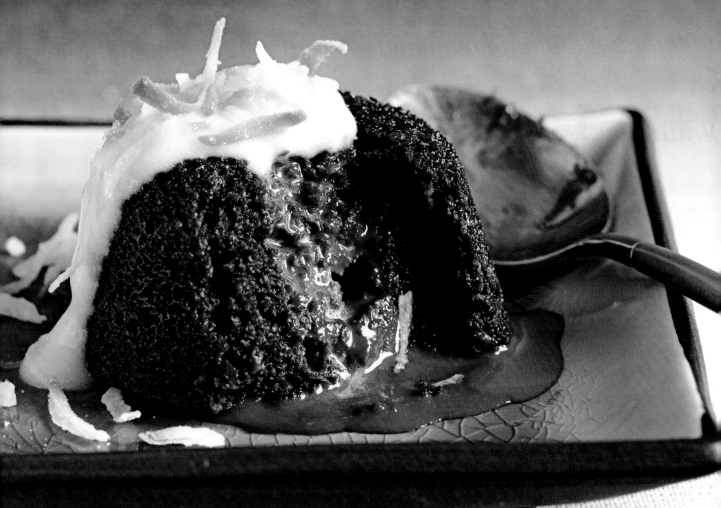

recipe index

continued on page 158

continued from page 157

recipe guide

See how we calculate nutrition information to help you count calories, carbs, and serving sizes.

Inside Our Recipes

Precise serving sizes (listed below the recipe title) help you to manage portions.

Ingredients listed as optional are not included in the per-serving nutrition analysis.

When kitchen basics such as ice, salt, black pepper, and nonstick cooking spray are not listed in the ingredients list, they are italicized in the directions.

Ingredients
• Tub-style vegetable oil spread refers to 60% to 70% vegetable oil product.
• Lean ground beef refers to 95% or leaner ground beef.

Nutrition Information

Nutrition facts per serving and food exchanges are noted with each recipe.

Test Kitchen tips and sugar substitutes are listed after the recipe directions.

When ingredient choices appear, we use the first one to calculate the nutrition analysis.

Key to Abbreviations

cal. = calories
sat. fat = saturated fat
chol. = cholesterol
carb. = carbohydrate
pro. = protein

metric information

The charts on this page provide a guide for converting measurements from the U.S. customary system, which is used throughout this book, to the metric system.

Product Differences

Most of the ingredients called for in the recipes in this book are available in most countries. However, some are known by different names. Here are some common American ingredients and their possible counterparts:

* All-purpose flour is enriched, bleached or unbleached white household flour. When self-rising flour is used in place of all-purpose flour in a recipe that calls for leavening, omit the leavening agent (baking soda or baking powder) and salt.
* Baking soda is bicarbonate of soda.
* Cornstarch is cornflour.
* Golden raisins are sultanas.
* Light-color corn syrup is golden syrup.
* Powdered sugar is icing sugar.
* Sugar (white) is granulated, fine granulated, or castor sugar.
* Vanilla or vanilla extract is vanilla essence.

Volume and Weight

The United States traditionally uses cup measures for liquid and solid ingredients. The chart below shows the approximate imperial and metric equivalents. If you are accustomed to weighing solid ingredients, the following approximate equivalents will be helpful.

* 1 cup butter, castor sugar, or rice = 8 ounces = $\frac{1}{2}$ pound = 250 grams
* 1 cup flour = 4 ounces = $\frac{1}{4}$ pound = 125 grams
* 1 cup icing sugar = 5 ounces = 150 grams

Canadian and U.S. volume for a cup measure is 8 fluid ounces (237 ml), but the standard metric equivalent is 250 ml.

1 British imperial cup is 10 fluid ounces.

In Australia, 1 tablespoon equals 20 ml, and there are 4 teaspoons in the Australian tablespoon.

Spoon measures are used for smaller amounts of ingredients. Although the size of the tablespoon varies slightly in different countries, for practical purposes and for recipes in this book, a straight substitution is all that's necessary. Measurements made using cups or spoons always should be level unless stated otherwise.

Common Weight Range Replacements

Imperial / U.S.	Metric
$\frac{1}{2}$ ounce	15 g
1 ounce	25 g or 30 g
4 ounces ($\frac{1}{4}$ pound)	115 g or 125 g
8 ounces ($\frac{1}{2}$ pound)	225 g or 250 g
16 ounces (1 pound)	450 g or 500 g
$1\frac{1}{4}$ pounds	625 g
$1\frac{1}{2}$ pounds	750 g
2 pounds or $2\frac{1}{4}$ pounds	1,000 g or 1 Kg

Oven Temperature Equivalents

Fahrenheit Setting	Celsius Setting*	Gas Setting
300°F	150°C	Gas Mark 2 (very low)
325°F	160°C	Gas Mark 3 (low)
350°F	180°C	Gas Mark 4 (moderate)
375°F	190°C	Gas Mark 5 (moderate)
400°F	200°C	Gas Mark 6 (hot)
425°F	220°C	Gas Mark 7 (hot)
450°F	230°C	Gas Mark 8 (very hot)
475°F	240°C	Gas Mark 9 (very hot)
500°F	260°C	Gas Mark 10 (extremely hot)
Broil	Broil	Grill

Electric and gas ovens may be calibrated using celsius. However, for an electric oven, increase celsius setting 10 to 20 degrees when cooking above 160°C. For convection or forced air ovens (gas or electric), lower the temperature setting 25°F/10°C when cooking at all heat levels.

Baking Pan Sizes

Imperial / U.S.	Metric
9x1$\frac{1}{2}$-inch round cake pan	22- or 23x4-cm (1.5 L)
9x1$\frac{1}{2}$-inch pie plate	22- or 23x4-cm (1 L)
8x8x2-inch square cake pan	20x5-cm (2 L)
9x9x2-inch square cake pan	22- or 23x4.5-cm (2.5 L)
11x7x1$\frac{1}{2}$-inch baking pan	28x17x4-cm (2 L)
2-quart rectangular baking pan	30x19x4.5-cm (3 L)
13x9x2-inch baking pan	34x22x4.5-cm (3.5 L)
15x10x1-inch jelly roll pan	40x25x2-cm
9x5x3-inch loaf pan	23x13x8-cm (2 L)
2-quart casserole	2 L

U.S. / Standard Metric Equivalents

$\frac{1}{8}$ teaspoon = 0.5 ml	
$\frac{1}{4}$ teaspoon = 1 ml	
$\frac{1}{2}$ teaspoon = 2 ml	
1 teaspoon = 5 ml	
1 tablespoon = 15 ml	
2 tablespoons = 25 ml	
$\frac{1}{4}$ cup = 2 fluid ounces = 50 ml	
$\frac{1}{3}$ cup = 3 fluid ounces = 75 ml	
$\frac{1}{2}$ cup = 4 fluid ounces = 125 ml	
$\frac{2}{3}$ cup = 5 fluid ounces = 150 ml	
$\frac{3}{4}$ cup = 6 fluid ounces = 175 ml	
1 cup = 8 fluid ounces = 250 ml	
2 cups = 1 pint = 500 ml	
1 quart = 1 litre	